Comments on *Eating Well for Kidney*

'I like the book and think it reads nicely. I'm sure it'll go down well.'

GEORGE HARTLEY, Chief Renal Dietitian,
Freeman Hospital, Newcastle-upon-Tyne

'This h   ild easily be used by anyone who wished to follow healthy
eatir   nes and was looking for some new inspirational meals. I
hav   ried out a few of the recipes and thoroughly enjoyed them.'

HELEN MILLAR, Specialist Diabetes Dietitian,
Glasgow

'As   nced renal dietitian, I highly recommend this book to people
w   ronic kidney disease. For those with more severe kidney
p   so recommend their companion book, *Eating Well with
Kid   .'

SUE PERRY, Chair of the Renal Nutrition Group
of the British Dietetic Association

'I am far   being a cook of any sort, but I have gone through the
recipes   clarity of the instructions is such that I would not be
deter   'having a go" . . . excellent!'

SIRAK SARGENT, London

'I ha   number of recipes that I would like to eat, and which are
fairl   nake . . . I would both buy the book and recommend it.'

PAUL SLATER, London

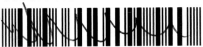

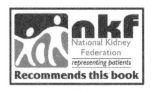

Recommends this book

Eating Well
for
Kidney Health

A practical guide and cookbook

Helena Jackson, BSc, PgDip, MSc, RD
Renal Dietitian, St George's Hospital, London

Claire Green, BSc, RD
Renal Dietitian, St George's Hospital, London

Gavin James, BSc, MSc, RD
Clinical Services Manager,
St George's Hospital, London

CLASS PUBLISHING · LONDON

Printing history
First published 2009

The authors and publishers welcome feedback from the users of this book. Please contact the publishers.

Class Publishing, Barb House, Barb Mews, London W6 7PA, UK
Telephone: 020 7371 2119
Fax: 020 7371 2878 [International +4420]
email: post@class.co.uk
www.class.co.uk

The information presented in this book is accurate and current to the best of the authors' knowledge. The authors and publisher, however, make no guarantee as to, and assume no responsibility for, the correctness, sufficiency or completeness of such information or recommendation. The reader is advised to consult a doctor regarding all aspects of individual health care.

A CIP catalogue record for this book is available from the British Library

ISBN 978 1 85959 2045

10 9 8 7 6 5 4 3 2 1

Edited by Richenda Milton-Thompson

Illustrations and artwork by David Woodroffe

Designed and typeset by Martin Bristow

Printed and bound in Finland by

Contents

Acknowledgements

The idea and support for this book came from Richard Warner who has a unique passion and drive in providing nutrition information for the wider public. We are also grateful to our editor, Richenda Milton-Thompson, for guiding us throughout the process with her customary wisdom, patience and understanding. Over much of the eighteen months, she has coped admirably with having three authors in entirely different places, geographically, professionally and domestically.

A special acknowledgment is due to Annie Cassidy for her extensive work on earlier drafts of several chapters in the present book. She was an invaluable co-author on our previous book and has had a most positive influence on this one.

We have been fortunate to have a number of expert professional and patient advisers who have helped us in planning, writing and reviewing the book. They have been so generous in giving their time to review the manuscript and the book has benefited enormously from their insightful comments and contributions. We are also very grateful to those people who contributed and tested recipes for the cookery section of the book and to those who have helped in other ways. Particular thanks go to Yajnik Bhageerutty, Naomi Cohen, Gillian Green, Michael Green, George Hartley, Sam Kanisius, Clare Jackson, Ronnie Jackson, Althea Mahon, Andrea McManus, Helen Millar, Freddy Rebello, Joe Ross, Sirak Sargent and Paul Slater.

We greatly appreciate the help and support of our renal and dietetic colleagues at St George's Hospital, London and at Middlemore Hospital, New Zealand. A heartfelt thanks also goes to our friends and families for their unstinting love, help and support. Without all of them, this book would have never been completed (although some of the younger members could have been a little more obliging at times).

Last, but not least, we are grateful for the invaluable experience gained through our work as renal dietitians in sharing the questions, knowledge and advice of people living with chronic kidney disease. They have informed us and inspired us in writing this book. We hope that, in return, we have succeeded in helping to make eating for health as easy and enjoyable for a far greater number of people than we, as clinicians, could ever hope to see.

Helena Jackson, Claire Green and Gavin James
London, 2009

Foreword

In February 2005 the Department of Health published The National Service Framework for Renal Services Part Two: Chronic Kidney Disease (CKD). Until that date, the only people identified with kidney disease were the 40,000 who had progressed right through to complete renal failure, and who could therefore survive only because of dialysis or a transplant. The National Service Framework was to change all this, making it the intention to identify and manage everyone with early stage kidney disease by means of blood tests in GP practices. It is thought that upwards of 3 million people might be identified in this way, suffering early stage chronic kidney disease, their condition being either stable or deteriorating.

A pattern is quickly emerging, picked up by the NKF Helpline, showing clearly that people who have been given this news by their GP want to do whatever they can to stabilise their condition and prevent deterioration toward end stage renal failure. It is all about living a healthier life and, in particular, eating in an appropriate way that helps not hinders the condition.

There is much that can be done. Some foods are quite harmful to kidneys, while others are undoubtedly beneficial. Kidneys do amazing work filtering and cleaning 200 litres of blood a day. If yours need a helping hand, this book will tell you how to look after them.

Food is a joy, restrictions can be tiresome. This book shows you how to 'bypass tiresome' and eat well!

Timothy F Statham OBE
Chief Executive
National Kidney Federation

Foreword

Food should be enjoyable, but if you've been found to have chronic kidney disease it can be difficult to know which foods are best to choose that will still taste great.

Healthy eating is an important part of the treatment for chronic kidney disease, as controlling your weight, blood pressure and diabetes all help to protect your kidneys. You need a reliable and informative source of expert advice to help you with your food choices. Dietitians can provide you with up-to-date personal advice but it can be difficult to find additional recipes and information specifically designed for people with chronic kidney disease.

All three authors are experienced registered renal dietitians and are well placed to provide this information. Using their expertise, they have produced practical, easy to follow advice and plenty of tasty recipes.

As an experienced renal dietitian, I highly recommend this book to people with early chronic kidney disease. For those with more severe kidney problems, I also recommend their companion book, *Eating Well with Kidney Failure*.

This book shows you that food can be both healthy and enjoyable!

Sue Perry BSc, Pg Dip, RD
Chair of the Renal Nutrition Group
of the British Dietetic Association

Introduction

This book is about eating, drinking and good food. It is full of quick, simple and great-tasting recipes for people with chronic kidney disease (CKD), along with their friends and families. Our focus is on healthy eating, and why this is so important in helping to manage CKD. We want to show those of you living with CKD that eating for health can be an easy and effective way to improve your chances of living long and active lives.

The advice in this book is broadly aimed at those people with mild to moderate CKD, categorised as CKD Stage 1 to 3, or for those with kidneys working up to 30% normal (see the Box below). People with more severe kidney disease and those needing dialysis are likely to require further or alternative advice. They may find the following book more helpful: *Eating Well with Kidney Failure* by Helena Jackson, Annie Cassidy and Gavin James. Full details of this and other useful resources are given in Appendix 1.

The five stages (categories) of chronic kidney disease (CKD)

Stage 1   Kidney damage with normal function

Stage 2   Kidney damage and slight decrease in kidney function

Stage 3   Moderate decrease in function – kidneys working at 30–59% normal

Stage 4   Severe decrease in function – kidneys working at only 15–29% normal

Stage 5   Established renal failure. Function of less than 15% normal. Approaching the need for/already on dialysis

---

Some people with kidney disease will have the opportunity to discuss what they eat with a dietitian. This book is not designed to replace this personal advice. Rather, it aims to help you be better informed when you see your doctor, dietitian or other health professionals. We hope that it will answer some questions that you may not think of or have time to ask in clinic, and that it will provide you with additional information and support.

The book is divided into two sections. The first gives some factual information about food and nutrition in relation to kidney disease. The second includes over 50 delicious recipes, to show you that eating can still be pleasurable. There are hints and tips on choosing and eating meals, including takeaways, pre-packaged meals and food for celebrations and special occasions.

As well as being tasty and simple to produce, the recipes have been chosen to help you to adapt favourite recipes and make them suitable for your particular diet. They have all been tried and tested – the finished dishes have been tasted by our friends, relatives, colleagues and patients. We are grateful for the help of all our 'tasters' in producing the end result.

Few of those with CKD will need to make drastic changes to what they eat. Reading this book will reassure some of you that your diet is fine as it is, or that small changes only are needed. A few readers, however, may benefit from making more changes to their diet. This will usually be either because they have other health problems, or because they wish to reduce the risk of developing such problems in the future. We hope that the recipes in this book will help those for whom this is a concern.

We have based this book on our experience as people who enjoy food, as well as our experience as dietitians working with people who have CKD. We hope that it will help you take control of this important aspect of your life, and use food in a way that successfully combines health and enjoyment.

Part 1 – FOOD FACTS

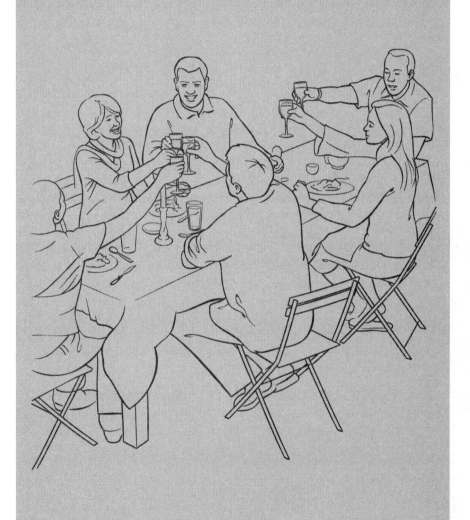

1
How can I protect my kidneys?

Most people with chronic kidney disease (CKD) and mildly reduced kidney function do not have symptoms and therefore do not know they have the condition. You may be at risk if you have diabetes or high blood pressure, or if a close member of your family has kidney disease. Your doctor can run a test to find out how well your kidneys are working.

Although it may be a shock to be told that you have kidney disease, there is plenty you can do to improve your health and help protect your kidneys from further damage. For example:

- achieve and maintain a healthy weight;
- achieve a good blood pressure (ask your doctor what you should aim for);
- if you have diabetes, aim for good diabetes control;
- reduce your risk from heart disease.

From the dietary perspective, this is surprisingly good news as all these health targets can be helped by a move towards a healthy, balanced diet, with an emphasis on reducing salt, to help control blood pressure. This means that you do not need to adopt strange, unusual or antisocial eating habits to have a kidney-friendly diet; but you do need to take healthy eating seriously. This will help you to control your weight, blood pressure, blood fats and sugars, and provide the protection against chronic diseases, including heart disease. Heart disease is the major cause of death for people with kidney disease, so eating to protect your heart is as important as protecting your kidneys.

Obviously this should not replace any medication or other intervention that your doctor recommends, but a kidney-friendly diet can also help some of the drugs work properly and, in the long term, help reduce the need for some drugs. For example, losing weight sensibly with a suitable diet and exercise can improve your overall health, as well as reducing blood fats, blood pressure and control of diabetes. So adopt a healthy lifestyle with a balanced diet, and you may find that your doctor is able to cut down on your tablets.

There is no single diet for kidney disease or reduced kidney function. Kidney disease may affect different people in different ways. Some people have fewer symptoms while others feel unwell from an early stage, sometimes due to other medical problems. Some symptoms can affect the ability and desire to eat. These range from feeling too tired to cook after a day's work, to experiencing taste changes, sickness and excessive weight loss. Often effort is needed to eat enough, rather than worrying about eating too much.

Other changes to diet may be needed in the early stages of CKD. Healthy kidneys control the level of water and minerals such as potassium, phosphate and sodium in the body. Reduced kidney function can disturb this balance. As these substances come from the diet, changes to food intake are sometimes needed to control their levels within the body.

It is important for everyone with CKD, or at risk of CKD, to discuss their condition and symptoms with their doctor. If diet is a particular issue, you may be referred on to a dietitian for further advice.

WHAT DOES A DIETITIAN DO?

A dietitian is an expert in nutrition, who will give individualised advice taking account of your particular dietary needs and preferences, as well as any additional religious, social, medical or dietary requirements that affect the foods that you can choose.

Not everyone who is diagnosed with chronic kidney disease will automatically see a specialist kidney (renal) dietitian as they are usually based within a kidney unit and tend to see people with more advanced disease. Some people may find that they will receive general dietary and lifestyle advice through their GP, practice nurse or through another hospital department such as the diabetes clinic. They will all be able to refer anyone who needs more individual advice to a local dietitian. A dietitian will advise you on four main aspects:

- A healthy diet (a well-balanced diet) that contains all the nutrients the body needs.

- Ways of preventing – or addressing – any other chronic (long-term) health problems such as diabetes, high blood pressure, heart disease and being overweight.

- The best foods to eat to control the build-up of waste products in the body.

- Ways of preventing – or addressing – any unintentional weight loss or malnutrition.

As you can see, this covers a wide range of topics relating to your nutritional health. The information in this book should help to back up the advice you receive from health professionals. It will also help you to take control of looking after your own kidneys and and overall health.

2
Energy

WHAT IS IT?

Everyone needs an adequate supply of energy for the body to function normally, for growth and replacement of tissue as well as any physical activity. If your weight is to be stable over time, your energy levels must be in balance, that is:

Energy taken in (as food or drink) = Energy used up (by activity/exercise)

If you eat more energy than your body needs, your body stores this extra energy as fat and you become overweight. If you eat less energy, your body will start to use up its reserves and you will lose weight. This happens, for example, if you 'go on a (weight-reducing) diet'. The change in weight will be due to loss of both muscle and fat. However, your aim is to lose any excess fat stores without losing any muscle. Raising activity levels can help to bring your energy levels back into balance, reduce fat stores and build up muscle stores. In other words, being more active will help to get rid of the flab and make you fitter and stronger.

WHAT HAPPENS IF YOUR KIDNEYS ARE NOT WORKING SO WELL?

Having kidney disease does not, in itself, change the amount of energy you need. This depends on your individual body function and make-up, how active you are, as well as on whether you have any other medical conditions.

It may be that you are overweight (see Chapter 10). If this is the case, your health is likely to be improved by losing some weight. This will reduce your risk of heart disease and cancer, and help to prevent and control conditions such as diabetes and high blood pressure. It is wise for anyone with a medical condition to check with their doctor before trying to lose weight (see Chapter 10, pages 42–48, for more information on weight control).

On the other hand, people sometimes find that it becomes more difficult to eat enough energy, perhaps because they have lost their appetite. This can be for a number of reasons, from anxiety to a worsening medical condition. Reduced energy intake can lead to ill health, muscle loss and nutritional deficiencies. If you feel that you are having trouble eating enough, or are losing weight without meaning to, you should ask to see a dietitian.

ENERGY IN THE DIET

The energy we get from food is measured in kilocalories (usually referred to simply as 'calories'), and varies depending on the different nutrients that the food contains (see the box below). Be aware that alcohol also contains calories.

Fat	9 (kilo) calories per gram
Carbohydrate (sugar and starches)	4 (kilo) calories per gram
Protein	4 (kilo) calories per gram
Alcohol	7 (kilo) calories per gram

Energy from fat

Fat is the most concentrated form of energy or calories. Weight for weight, it has over twice the energy of carbohydrates or protein. It is important to know this if you need to gain or lose weight. This is the theory behind low-fat diets; they cut out fat and use reduced-fat products to lower the total number of calories you eat. Eating fewer fatty foods, such as butter, margarine, oil or full-fat products such as full-cream milk and replacing them with skimmed milk, low-fat and diet yoghurts, can help. Other examples of fatty foods to reduce include cream, pastry and fried foods. The type of fat that you eat has an influence on your risk of heart disease. The better choices are the unsaturated fats and oils, such as rapeseed (often sold as 'vegetable' oil) and olive oils and margarines. These should replace the saturated fats, such as ghee, butter, palm oil or lard.

If you are underweight, or have a poor appetite and are unable to increase the amount of food you can eat, you may want your diet to be richer in energy. In this case you can include fatty foods in your diet but where possible try to choose the unsaturated types of fat to increase in your diet. For more information about fats, see Chapter 4.

| Some examples of starchy and sugary foods ||
Starchy foods	Sugars/sugary foods
Bread	Sucrose
Potato	Glucose
Rice	Fructose
Pasta	White sugar
Noodles	Brown sugar
Yam	Demerara sugar
Breakfast cereals (plain)	Honey
Plantain	Maltodextrins
Chapatti	Molasses
Polenta	Jam, jelly, marmalade
Couscous	Sweets (boiled, chews, mints, etc.)
Oats	Turkish delight
	Full sugar fizzy drinks and squash

Energy from carbohydrates

There are two types of carbohydrates, starches and sugars (see the table above). As well as being a good source of energy, starchy foods can be naturally low in fat and provide many essential nutrients such as B vitamins and some protein. Wholegrain varieties also provide fibre to prevent constipation and tend to be more filling. Sugar, however, is found mainly in processed foods such as sweets, cakes and fizzy drinks, which don't have many other nutrients. Eating too many sugary foods and snacks can lead to health problems including overweight and tooth decay.

Generally, the recommendation is to take most of your energy in the form of high-fibre, starchy foods such as wholemeal bread and pasta, brown rice and wholegrain cereals. It is also beneficial to eat less sugary foods, especially if you are trying to lose weight. Ways to reduce your sugar intake can be seen in the table opposite.

People who need to put on weight are sometimes advised to include some sugary foods, such as biscuits or desserts, because they tend to be high in calories and not very filling. Check with your doctor or dietitian if you feel this applies to you, especially if you have diabetes.

Foods high and low in sugar	
Higher sugar choices	**Lower sugar choices**
Standard squashes and fizzy drinks	Diet, low-calorie, 'sugar-free', 'no added sugar' drinks/squashes/fizzy drinks
Sucrose Add sugar/jam/honey/syrup to foods and drinks	Choose artificial sweeteners e.g. Canderel/Hermesetas/Sweetex or shop's own brand of saccharin-based or aspartame-based sweetener for desserts and drinks
Standard yoghurts (Note: low-fat yoghurts may still be high in sugar)	Diet or 'lite' yoghurts
Fruit tinned in syrup	Fruit tinned in fruit juice (Note: these may need to be drained if you are on a low-potassium diet)
Standard milk puddings and desserts	Reduced-sugar desserts
Sugar-coated or cream-filled biscuits	Plain biscuits e.g. rich tea or wholemeal biscuits
Sugar-coated breakfast cereals	Plain cereals e.g. Weetabix, Shredded Wheat, cornflakes, porridge

Carbohydrate-rich foods can also be categorised by their glycaemic index (GI). This measures the rate at which they are broken down to produce glucose (the sugar found in blood). Foods, such as wholegrain breads and cereals, oats, pulses and pasta, have a lower GI and cause a more gradual rise in blood glucose. This is preferable to the rapid rise (and fall) in blood sugar caused by high glycaemic foods such as sweet drinks, white bread and sugary breakfast cereals.

It can help to choose a lower GI food instead of its higher GI equivalent as long as you are sticking to healthy eating guidelines. Think about GI as a positive message to include more wholegrain cereals and bread, pasta, noodles, pulses and oats as well as fruit and vegetables. All fruits and vegetables have health benefits regardless of their GI rating. Some foods with a higher GI can still be included in a healthy diet. Examples might include white bread, pumpkin or unsalted rice crackers.

Mixing low GI foods into a higher GI dish can reduce the overall GI of the meal; for example, you could add lentils to the minced meat mixture in a shepherd's pie. Some of the recipes in this book have been chosen to show you how easy it is to include some healthy lower GI foods within your diet.

Some healthy lower GI foods

- Oat cereals, e.g. porridge, muesli (no added sugar)

- Granary/multigrain bread, pitta bread, ryebread

- Pasta, noodles, basmati rice, long grain white rice, bulgar wheat, pearl barley, semolina

- Yam, cassava, sweet potato, new potatoes

- Peas, dahls, lentils, most beans including chickpeas and baked beans (choose low-salt variety)

- Apples, oranges, pears, peaches, strawberries

3
Protein

WHAT IS IT?

Protein is important for normal function, growth and repair of all parts of the body, including the skin, muscles, blood and internal organs. Milk, meat, fish, eggs and soya beans are all rich in protein. Many other foods, such as bread, pasta, beans, nuts, lentils and peas, contain protein in smaller amounts.

Proteins are made up of smaller units called amino acids. Different proteins contain different amino acids. Some of these can be made by the body; but others, known as 'essential amino acids', cannot. This is why it is important to eat a variety of protein-containing foods to make sure that you get all of the amino acids you need.

WHAT HAPPENS IF YOUR KIDNEYS ARE NOT WORKING SO WELL?

Healthy kidneys get rid of the waste products of protein in the urine. When your kidneys are not working well, the level of urea and similar waste products can rise in your body. Many people have no symptoms from this, particularly in the earlier stages of chronic kidney disease (CKD). In more advanced CKD, a rise in these waste products may make people lose their appetite and feel unwell. Kidney failure can also cause the body to become less efficient at using protein from the diet.

HOW MUCH PROTEIN SHOULD YOU EAT?

Most people with chronic kidney disease need to eat a moderate amount of protein. In practice, this will generally mean including a modest portion of protein-rich food at two meals each day and avoiding high-protein drinks (limit milk to no more than one pint daily) and high-protein snacks. Limiting high-protein foods such as cheese and meat products has the extra benefits of lowering salt and fat intake. The actual amount of protein needed depends on body size and individual circumstances.

There are some people with CKD who may be advised to eat more protein-rich foods. This can be because their CKD is more advanced and causing poor appetite, or because their particular medical condition requires it.

Some kidney specialists think people with CKD should follow a low-protein diet because this will slow down the rate at which the kidneys fail. They also think that a low-protein diet will help to reduce the build-up of some of the toxic waste products normally dealt with by the kidneys. Other experts do not agree. They are also concerned that a low-protein diet is too restrictive for most people to follow and may lead to malnutrition in the long term. If you would like to find out more about the advantages and disadvantages of restricting protein in your diet, talk to your doctor or a dietitian.

PROTEIN IN THE DIET

☑ TRUE OR ☒ FALSE?

I need to eat meat to get enough protein in my diet.

☒ **FALSE.** Vegetarians can get all the protein they need by choosing a good variety of foods and eating a balanced diet.

What sort of food is best to eat?
Food that contains the most protein, with the full range of amino acids, tends to come from animals – for example, meat, chicken, fish, eggs, milk and cheese. Some vegetarian foods (such as quorn and tofu) are also rich in protein. Beans, lentils, pulses, nuts and some starchy foods also contain protein, but it is less concentrated and will be missing one or more essential amino acids. This means that vegetarians (and particularly vegans) have to take care to choose a range of protein-rich foods to make sure that they eat enough protein of the right kind.

Examples of vegetarian/vegan meals containing a good combination of protein foods

✱ a chickpea curry served with rice
✱ baked beans on toast
✱ wheat noodles with stir-fried tofu

It is worth noting that some dietary restrictions, such as low-potassium, low-phosphate and low-fat regimens can lead to a degree of protein restriction in the diet. See a dietitian for advice for balancing your protein needs with any dietary restrictions. There is more information on potassium in Chapter 6 and on phosphate in Chapter 7.

Healthy eating protein choices

Lean meat Trim visible fat and try baking, grilling or stewing with only the minimum added fat or oil. Naturally low in salt.

Poultry Remove the skin. Grill or roast instead of frying. Naturally low in salt.

Fish Aim for 2 portions weekly, one of which should be oily (e.g. salmon, trout, mackerel etc.) White fish (such as pollock, cod, whiting) is very low in fat. Grilled or baked instead of breaded, battered, fried. Tinned in spring water instead of brine. Avoid salted and smoked fish.
See www.fishonline.org for information on sustainable fish sources.

Eggs Boiled, poached etc., rather than fried. Naturally low in salt. Limit to about 4 per week if your blood cholesterol or phosphate levels are high.

Milk Choose semi-skimmed or skimmed. No more than 1 pint daily (includes milk in cooking and other foods) to limit protein and phosphate intake, unless advised otherwise.

Cheese and milk products Choose low fat/diet varieties of cheese, yoghurt etc. Low-fat cottage cheese and cream cheese are lower-salt choices.

Vegetarian alternatives Ingredients such as tofu and Quorn are, convenient and low fat. Watch out for added salt and fat in ready made products such as burgers, grills, ready meals etc.

Beans, lentils, pulses Wide choice, cheap, naturally low in fat and salt, low GI and high in valuable fibre. Can buy tinned in water or low salt/sugar baked beans for convenience. Add a handful or two of dried lentils to meat/vegetable dishes such as curry, stews etc.

High protein supplements

High protein supplements are widely available in health food shops, gyms and other outlets, but may be harmful to people with chronic kidney disease (see also page 38). You should check with your doctor or dietitian before taking any of these products.

4
Fats

WHAT IS FAT?

Dietary fat is the most energy-rich of all the nutrients we eat. Fats play a major role in increasing cholesterol levels in the body and can contribute to weight gain. However eliminating all fat from our diet is impractical, unhealthy and unnecessary. Fat is essential in bile and hormone production, insulation of organs and absorption of vitamins. We all need some fat in the diet, but it is important to eat the right kind of fats in the right quantities.

WHAT HAPPENS IF YOUR KIDNEYS ARE NOT WORKING SO WELL?

Heart disease is the major cause of death for people with kidney disease. It is important to think about keeping your heart healthy by eating less fat and controlling your cholesterol.

WHAT IS CHOLESTEROL?

The liver makes cholesterol from the saturated fats we eat. The cholesterol is carried around our bodies by proteins called lipoproteins. There are two types of lipoproteins: low density lipoproteins (LDL) and high density lipoproteins (HDL).

LDLs are often referred to as the 'bad' cholesterol; they take cholesterol from the liver to the body's cells. If there is a high level in your body it can

> ## ☑ TRUE OR ☒ FALSE?
>
> My cholesterol is high so I need to cut out cholesterol from my diet.
>
> ☒ FALSE. Dietary cholesterol does not generally have a strong influence on blood cholesterol. The type and amount of the fat in the diet is more important.

build up on the walls of your arteries causing narrowing, and restricting blood flow.

HDLs are often referred to as 'good' cholesterol; they take cholesterol away from the arteries to the liver to be eliminated from the body. This means that we need to aim for a low LDL level and a high HDL level.

Triglycerides are another type of fat found in the blood. People with high triglyceride levels are at increased risk of heart disease and stroke. The risk is greater in people who already have high cholesterol, diabetes or high blood pressure. People who eat a lot of fatty and/or sugary foods, or drink too much alcohol, are more likely to have raised triglyceride levels.

**Target cholesterol levels
(British Heart Foundation Guidelines)**

Total cholesterol under 4 mmols/L

LDL under 2 mmols/L

HDL above 1 mmol/L

Triglycerides under 1.7 mmols/L

What causes high cholesterol?
Two types of factors contribute to high cholesterol, firstly things you can do nothing to change and, secondly, factors over which you have some control.

Things you cannot change

- Gender – men tend to have higher cholesterol levels than women until the menopause. After this, the risks are equal.

- Age – Cholesterol increases with age.

- Ethnicity – Higher risk for some ethnicities e.g. Indo-Asian, Afro-Caribbean.

- Family history – if your family is affected by high cholesterol it is likely you will be as well.

Things you can change

- Your weight and shape (see Chapter 10).

- Your level of physical activity (Chapter 10).

- Your stress levels.

- Whether or not you smoke.

- Your diet (especially saturated and trans fats).

- The amount of alcohol you drink (see page 42).

WHAT ARE THE DIFFERENT TYPES OF FAT?

Saturated fats
It is important to reduce the amount of saturated fat in your diet.

This is the main cause of increased levels of 'bad' cholesterol (LDL). LDL increases the risk of fatty deposits in your arteries. It is mainly found in animal products e.g. meat products, cheese, butter, cream, lard, ghee, coconut oil, palm oil.

Polyunsaturated fats
These can help lower total cholesterol levels, but also tend to reduce the amount of 'good' HDL cholesterol. They are mainly found in corn, sunflower or soya oil, nuts and seeds (walnuts, pine nuts, sesame seeds and sunflower seeds). Oily fish contain a particular type of polyunsaturated fat called omega-3. This is believed to be helpful in improving cardiovascular health by decreasing the triglycerides, helping to reduce blood clots and inflammation. You should aim to eat at least 2 portions of fish a week, of which at least one should be oily.

Monounsaturated fats
These can lower the amounts of LDL without affecting the levels of HDL. They should replace the saturated fat in the diet. However monounsaturated fats still contain the same number of calories and will contribute to weight gain. Monounsaturated fats are found in olive oil, rapeseed oil (supermarket 'vegetable' oils are often made from rapeseed), avocado, nuts and seeds (almonds, cashews, hazelnuts, peanuts).

Trans fats
It is important to reduce the amount of trans fat in your diet. These fats have a similar effect to saturated fats by increasing 'bad' cholesterol. Trans fats, which are formed when vegetable oils are hydrogenated (artificially

hardened), cannot be digested by the body. They are used to make hard margarines and processed foods such as some cakes, biscuits and pastries.

Choosing the right fat

- Reduce the amount of saturated fat and replace with monounsaturated fats. Try olive or rapeseed oils and spreads instead of butter, ghee or lard.

- Reduce the total amount of fat you eat, especially if you are overweight. Try eating fewer biscuits, cakes and crisps and replace with more fruit or vegetables or low-fat starchy foods e.g. bread, rice, pasta, potatoes.

- Cut down on foods containing trans fats – including processed foods such as biscuits, cakes and pastries.

5
Salt (sodium)

WHAT IS IT?

Salt is the name commonly used for 'sodium chloride', which is naturally found in some foods and is added to others to add flavour and preserve them. Sodium is a part of salt, and is important in our bodies for fluid balance and blood pressure control, as well as ensuring our muscles and nerves work properly.

HOW MUCH SALT DO WE NEED?

Although salt is important for the body to function, we only need a very small amount. Currently in the UK, we eat an average of around 10 grams (the equivalent of two teaspoons) of salt every day. For good health it would be better to cut this to no more than 6 g of salt (2.5 g sodium) each day for adults and less for children.

WHY REDUCE YOUR SALT INTAKE?

Eating less salt can prevent or treat high blood pressure (hypertension) which will protect against strokes, heart attacks and further damage to the kidneys. It is also thought to reduce the risk of developing stomach cancer and bone disease.

Cutting down on salt can also help to prevent fluid retention which is sometimes a problem for people who have chronic kidney disease (CKD).

HOW CAN YOU REDUCE THE AMOUNT OF SALT YOU EAT?

Reducing the amount of salt you eat may make food taste bland at first, but after about 6–8 weeks, your taste buds will adjust to it. You will start tasting the food itself, rather than just the salt. If you speak to other people who have cut down on salt, they often say that they now dislike the taste of salty foods and prefer foods made with less salt.

There are three main ways to reduce your salt intake:

- Eat fewer processed foods and fewer foods that are naturally high in salt;

- Do not add salt at the table;

- Use less salt in cooking – try herbs, spices and other flavourings instead.

EATING FEWER SALTY FOODS

Surprisingly most of the salt we eat is hidden in processed foods. This accounts for three quarters of our total intake. Only one quarter of the salt we eat comes from the salt we add either at the table or in cooking.

Eating less of these types of food will help to cut down on salt in your diet. Fortunately, there is usually a lower-salt food that you can try instead. (See the table opposite.)

☑ *TRUE OR* ☒ *FALSE?*

Food labelled as having 'no added salt' means it is low in salt.

☒ **FALSE.** This term just means no salt has been added in the cooking process. It does not always mean that it is low in salt.
Other labelling terms are:
Reduced sodium Means it is at least 25 per cent lower in sodium than the standard product. The food could still be high in sodium, e.g. low-sodium soy sauce is lower in sodium than standard soy sauce, but it is still very salty.
Low in sodium Means a sodium content of less than 0.04 g per 100 g of food. This is a 'genuinely' low-salt food.

Working out whether foods are high in salt?

Many processed foods contain a high level of salt, so it is important to check food labels. This can be a bit confusing. At the moment many food labels state only the amount of sodium in the food. Some manufacturers may include the salt content, sometimes called the 'salt equivalent'. To compare the salt content of different foods, look for the 'sodium per 100 g' value on the label. If the salt content is stated you can also use that but

Reducing your intake of salty foods

Eat less	Choose instead
Processed and cured meats e.g. ham, bacon, sausages and tinned meats	Plain roast or grilled meat – cooked without added salt
Smoked fish Tinned fish in brine	Unsmoked fresh or frozen fish Tinned fish in spring water
Ready made, tinned, packet or instant soups. Meat and vegetable extracts such as Marmite, Bovril and Oxo	Homemade soup with water, spices and herbs or other flavourings Low-salt stock cubes
Salted snacks such as crisps, salted peanuts, Bombay mix, chevra	Low-salt crackers, rice cakes or crisps, plain unsalted popcorn
Bottled sauces e.g. ketchup, salad cream, Worcester sauce, soya sauce	Try olive oil, vinegar or homemade French dressing. Low-sodium soya sauce (contains about one-third less salt)
Cheese – including Cheddar, blue cheeses, Parmesan, Edam etc.	Cottage cheese, ricotta and cream cheese
Tinned vegetables in brine	Use fresh or frozen vegetables or those tinned in water
Pickles, stock cubes, salted flavourings	Herbs, spices, salt-free stock cubes and seasoning mixes

make sure you are comparing like for like (salt with salt or sodium with sodium) as it is easy to mix up the two.

The salt content of foods can vary, as shown in the table overleaf. You also need to think about the size of the portions you are eating. Adults should try to eat no more than 6 g salt (2.5 g sodium) each day.

Next time you go shopping, compare the labels on different foods, to help you choose those that are lower in salt. Look at the figure for salt or sodium per 100 g. To convert from sodium to salt, multiply the amount by 2.5. If the amount per 10 g is between 0.5 g sodium (1.3 g salt) and 0.1 g sodium (0.3 g salt), this indicates a medium level of sodium.

Comparison of sodium contents in different foods *What is 'a lot'? What is 'a little'?*			
A LOT (More than 0.5 g sodium/100 g)		**A LITTLE** (Less than 0.1 g sodium/100 g)	
Food	**Grams (g) sodium per 100 g food**	**Food**	**Grams (g) sodium per 100 g food**
Salad cream	1.1	Vinegar	0.02
Cornflakes	1.0	Shredded Wheat	Less than 0.01
Corned beef	0.9	Roast beef	0.05
Cream crackers	0.6	Matzo crackers	Less than 0.01
Baked beans	0.5	Frozen green peas	Less than 0.01

DO NOT ADD SALT AT THE TABLE

Try to get out of the habit of adding salt to food at the table, especially if you tend to do so without even tasting it first. Watch for hidden salt in many sauces and condiments such as tomato ketchup, mustard, soy sauce, chutney, pickles and brown sauce. To help keep your salt intake down, try to use these sparingly or avoid them altogether.

Again, check food labels and look for the low-salt alternatives, such as vinegar, cranberry sauce, mint sauce, homemade mustard (from mustard powder) or homemade salad dressing (see recipes). If you can't do without soy sauce, try the lower sodium version which is about one third less salty.

Salt substitutes
You may have come across salt substitutes that are promoted as healthy alternatives to salt. Some of these such as 'LoSalt', 'Selora' or 'Ruthmol', are made with potassium, and are NOT suitable for people with kidney

disease and a number of other health problems. Check with your doctor before using them.

REDUCE SALT IN COOKING

Try to cook with fresh food as often as possible rather than using ready-made or convenience foods or sauces. If you do use manufactured products for part of the meal, cook the pasta, rice, vegetables or other accompaniments without salt to compensate. Use more herbs (dried, fresh or frozen), garlic, black pepper or other spices and flavourings such as lemon juice. Remember that many manufactured flavourings can be high in salt, for example garlic or celery salt, sea salt, curry pastes and seasoning powders such as Cajun seasoning or tandoori powder. Look out for salt-free curry powder or spice mixtures, seasonings and stock cubes.

You can experiment with herbs, spices and other flavourings to boost the taste of your food without relying on salt. Here are a few ideas for tasty combinations of flavourings with some familiar foods.

Using herbs and spices to flavour foods	
Roast meat	Apple with pork, mustard or pepper with beef, tarragon with chicken, rosemary with lamb
Grills	Flavoured oil, lemon juice, garlic, honey, coriander
Mince/stews	Bouquet garni, bayleaf, basil, oregano, sage, cumin, garam masala
Fish	Parsley, dill, fresh coriander, vinegar, lemon or lime juice, turmeric, lemon grass
Potatoes	Mint, garlic, chopped chives, spring onions, bayleaf
Vegetables	Basil, oregano, chives, thyme, parsley

6
Potassium

WHAT IS IT?

Potassium (the symbol 'K' is often used) is a mineral that is vital for life. The level in the body is normally controlled by the kidneys. This is important for the normal function of all nerves and muscles, including the heart. Potassium is present in a wide variety of foods including fruit, vegetables, meat and milk.

WHAT HAPPENS IF YOUR KIDNEYS ARE NOT WORKING SO WELL?

When kidneys are not functioning well they may lose the ability to fully control potassium levels. This can lead to a blood potassium level which is above or below the usual range of 3.5–5.0 mmol/L. (Your hospital may use a slightly different normal range, so do check this locally.) High potassium levels (hyperkalaemia) can interfere with normal muscle and nerve function and cause the heart to beat irregularly. Low potassium levels (hypokalaemia) can also cause problems.

DO YOU NEED A LOW-POTASSIUM DIET?

If your potassium level is normal, you won't need a low-potassium diet. This is the case with most people with chronic kidney disease (CKD) in its early stages. If your potassium level is too high, it can be controlled by reducing the amount of potassium you eat. Your doctor can refer you to a dietitian for a proper assessment of your diet to help you cut down on potassium without losing out on taste or any important nutrients.

OTHER CAUSES OF ABNORMAL POTASSIUM LEVELS

A high potassium level may not always be caused by diet. Other factors include drugs such as ACE inhibitors (a type of blood pressure tablet), constipation, muscle breakdown, blood transfusions and poorly controlled diabetes. Low potassium levels can also occur with certain diuretics (water tablets) as well as a low dietary intake of potassium.

CHOOSING A LOW-POTASSIUM DIET

Which foods contain potassium?
Most food contains potassium. If you need to eat less potassium, you will be advised to limit certain high-potassium foods or avoid them altogether. High-potassium foods include coffee, chocolate, dried fruit, bananas, fruit juices and vegetable juices. Some foods, such as milk and certain fruits and vegetables, contain a moderate level of potassium and provide other important nutrients. Your dietitian will give you information on the amounts and types of these foods that you can eat. There are also many foods that are low in potassium and which can be eaten freely or as usual, such as tea, bread, rice, pasta and noodles.

Choosing and adapting recipes
The recipes in this book are not specifically designed for a low-potassium diet. They have been chosen to help you increase your fruit and vegetable intake, rather than limit it. However, if you are on a low-potassium diet you should be able to include most of the dishes in your diet or adapt them using the tips throughout the book.

Food labelling
Potassium isn't usually listed on food labels. If you need to follow a low-potassium diet you can check the ingredient list on the packet so that you can avoid items containing a lot of ingredients that are high in potassium. You should avoid any foods labelled as containing salt substitutes such as LoSalt, Ruthmol, etc. These may be used in products advertising themselves as 'low in salt' or 'low in sodium', but they do contain a lot of potassium. (For more information on food labelling, see pages 62–66.)

The potassium diet – first steps
Do NOT restrict your potassium intake unless you are advised to do so. Many high-potassium foods, such as fruit and vegetables, are an important part of a healthy diet.

If you have been advised by your doctor to eat less potassium, you should ask to see your local dietitian for advice on your own particular diet and medical condition. In the meantime there are a few general changes that can help to reduce potassium intake.

Tips for reducing your potassium intake
(Only if advised to do so by a health professional)

- Choose lower potassium drinks such as water, tea (black or herbal), squash, spirits, dry white wine, instead of higher potassium alternatives such as fruit juice, vegetable juices, smoothies, coffee, chocolate drinks, fortified wines, cider etc.

- Choose lower potassium snacks such as plain biscuits, cakes, crumpets, crackers, boiled sweets and mints instead of higher potassium choices such as chocolate, toffee, crisps, nuts, Bombay mix.

- Potassium dissolves in water. Cooking methods such as steaming, microwaving, baking, roasting and frying use very little or no water and do not remove potassium. So try to boil your vegetables and potatoes before eating, baking, roasting or adding to stews, curries, soups or otherwise cooking further.

- Moderate your fruit and vegetable intake – keep to a maximum of five (approximately 80 g) portions each day. Fresh, frozen and tinned (without salt) are fine, but reduce dried fruit and dried vegetables.

- Avoid salt substitutes such as LoSalt, Ruthmol, etc. Use more herbs, spices and other flavourings.

7
Phosphate

WHAT IS IT?

Phosphate (the symbol PO_4 is often used) is a form of the mineral phosphorous and is needed to help make, maintain and repair your bones. The kidneys normally control the amount of phosphate in the body. If you eat too much phosphate, you will get rid of it in your urine whereas, if you aren't eating enough, your kidneys will reduce the amount that you lose. In this way, the level of phosphate in your blood is regulated.

Phosphate is mainly found in protein-rich foods such as meat, fish, milk, cheese, eggs, yoghurt and nuts.

WHAT HAPPENS IF YOUR KIDNEYS ARE NOT WORKING SO WELL?

As kidney disease progresses, the kidneys lose their ability to control phosphate levels in the body. This can result in an increase in blood phosphate levels above the normal range of 0.8–1.4 mmol/L (your hospital laboratory may use a slightly different normal range, so do check this locally).

This change in phosphate control can stimulate the production of a hormone called parathyroid hormone (PTH). If too much PTH is produced, this will cause damage to bones and blood vessels over time. Chronic kidney disease (CKD) also reduces your body's ability to make a useable form of vitamin D, and will contribute to this effect (see Chapter 9). People with CKD are often prescribed a special vitamin D supplement, such as alphacalcidol, which does not rely on the kidneys for its action in the body.

DO YOU NEED A LOW-PHOSPHATE DIET?

You should not attempt to follow a low-phosphate diet unless advised by a kidney specialist doctor (nephrologist) or dietitian.

Most people with mild to moderate kidney disease are able to control their blood phosphate levels and will not be advised to go on any specific diet. For this reason, we have chosen not to mark our recipes in this book for phosphate content.

On the other hand, there is some evidence that it may be prudent for people with CKD to avoid a diet that is high in phosphate. By following the healthy eating guidelines and not eating excessive amounts of protein you will control your phosphate intake anyway. However, here are some points to consider within your healthy eating plan, providing you have no loss of appetite or other relevant problems.

Limiting the phosphate content of your diet

- Limit milk to no more than 1 pint daily, including that used in cereals, desserts and other dishes.

- Avoid high protein snacks between meals, including nuts, meat samosas, fish cakes and other meat or fish products.

- Limit cheese, especially as snacks. This will also help you control your calorie, fat, salt and protein intake. Low-fat cottage cheese and cream cheese are useful choices.

- Reduce cola drinks. Try some alternative soft drinks such as lemonade, squash or flavoured waters.

If your kidney disease continues to progress, the levels of phosphate in your blood may start to rise. At this point, most people need to reduce the amount of phosphate they eat. If you are in this position, you should ask to see a dietitian for advice on your own particular diet and medical condition. This may involve limiting certain phosphate-rich foods such as milk, eggs, nuts and shellfish. In the meantime you can try following the points in the box above. You may also be asked to start taking phosphate-binding tablets with your food. These tablets combine with the food in your gut to remove some of the phosphate before it is taken up by your body.

8
Fluid balance

WHAT IS IT?

Healthy kidneys balance the level of fluid (water) in your body. They remove excess fluid in the body in the form of urine. Most people know that if they drink several additional cups of tea or glasses of water they will find themselves passing more urine than usual. This urine will probably be very dilute or light in colour. Conversely, if you drink less than usual, or get very hot and sweaty, your body will become dry or dehydrated, your kidneys will produce less urine and it will be more concentrated or darker in colour.

WHAT HAPPENS IF YOUR KIDNEYS ARE NOT WORKING SO WELL?

If kidney disease progresses the kidneys may lose some of their ability to balance the level of fluid in the body. This may lead to fluid (water) retention. Too much water within the body can cause unpleasant side effects and lead to heart problems in the longer term. Too little water (dehydration) also causes problems such as low blood pressure and dizziness.

If you think that you have any of the symptoms of fluid overload (see the box below), you should report them to your medical team.

> ### Some symptoms of fluid overload
>
> ✳ Fluid-related weight gain
>
> ✳ Ankle swelling and oedema (water in the skin)
>
> ✳ Shortness of breath (due to water around the lungs)
>
> ✳ Raised blood pressure
>
> ✳ Damage to the heart in the long term

HOW TO KEEP YOUR FLUID BALANCE RIGHT

Most people should aim for a good fluid intake, approximately 2 litres a day, particularly in conditions that increase sweating, such as hot weather and exercise.

If you do need to restrict your intake, you will be told how much you can drink each day. The amount will vary between individuals, and may change over time (see the box below), so it is important to review your fluid allowance regularly with your doctor. If you need to restrict your fluid intake do make sure to keep your salt intake under control (See Chapter 5). This will not only help you get rid of extra body water, but also prevent you becoming too thirsty and make it much easier to keep to your fluid restriction.

Factors affecting your fluid allowance

- The amount of urine you pass each day (this may change over time).

- Any period of illness.

- Certain medications (especially diuretics or 'water tablets').

Remember that changes in fluid status can sometimes hide changes in body (flesh) weight. So sometimes it is hard to work out whether your weight is changing due to changes in the fluid in your body or whether it is due to changes in flesh weight (the amount of fat or muscle you have). If any weight gain is due to fluid retention, you may feel fatter but do not cut back on your overall food intake as this will leave you short of energy and nutrients. Instead follow your doctor's advice on medication and salt and fluid control.

WHAT COUNTS AS FLUID?

If you have been advised to reduce your fluid intake, all liquids in your diet need to be counted as part of your fluid allowance. These include tea, water, alcohol and milk on cereals. Your allowance also includes foods that contain a lot of fluid, such as gravy, soup, sauces, jelly and ice-cream.

Handy fluid measures

One teacup = 150 mls

One small wine glass = 125 mls

One mug = 250 mls

Average can of fizzy drink = 330 mls

One pint = 560 mls

9
Vitamins, minerals and supplements

There are national government guidelines for vitamin, mineral and trace element requirements in health. However, very little is known about requirements in people who have chronic kidney disease (CKD). In general, a varied balanced diet should provide most of the nutrients that you need without supplements. If your appetite is poor you may feel that you should have a vitamin supplement. However, you may also need advice on eating enough energy, protein and other nutrients rather than simply focusing on supplementing one or more vitamin or mineral. So it is worth seeking some professional advice first.

If you take any vitamin or mineral supplements, herbal remedies or anything else that your doctor hasn't told you to take, it is important to let your doctor, pharmacist and dietitian know when you see them. Some can cause unpleasant side effects for people with kidney disease or other medical conditions. They may react badly when taken with your other medications, preventing them from working properly and making you feel ill. Or they may contain substances that only healthy kidneys can cope with properly.

VITAMINS

Vitamins are essential for health, and your body needs them in order to function properly. Eating a balanced diet (see pages 39–42) will help you get enough vitamins from your diet without the need for additional supplements.

There are two main categories of vitamins, those that are water-soluble (see table opposite) and those that are fat-soluble (see table on page 36).

Among the fat-soluble vitamins, vitamin A supplements are unlikely to be needed as this vitamin is retained in the body by people who have reduced kidney function.

Vitamin D is particularly important as it is usually made in the body from the action of sunlight on the skin, with the help of the kidneys. Some

Water-soluble vitamins		
Name	Function	Dietary sources
B1	Needed to convert food into energy	Breakfast cereals, bread, meat, dairy produce, vegetables
B2	Needed for growth and healthy body tissues, skin, eyes and nervous system	Milk, dairy produce, meat and cereals
Niacin	Needed to convert food into energy	Meat, dairy produce, breakfast cereals, bread, vegetables
B6	Helps the body to make use of protein	Cereal, meat, potatoes, milk and dairy produce
Folic acid	Helps the body to make use of protein and build healthy cells	Cereals, vegetables, meat, milk and dairy produce
B12	Needed for healthy blood cells and nerves	Meat, dairy produce, breakfast cereals, fish, eggs
C	Antioxidant, helps to protect cells and aids wound healing	Vegetables, potatoes, fruit, fruit juices

people, such as those living in a care home, who are housebound or who have very little exposure to sunlight for any other reason, may need standard vitamin D supplements. A special vitamin D supplement (e.g. alphacalcidol), which contains the active form of vitamin D, is prescribed for those people with CKD whose kidneys are losing the ability to make their own.

MINERALS

Minerals are an essential part of a balanced diet. They can be divided into two groups: minerals we require in relatively large quantities and others, known as trace elements, which are needed in only very small amounts. Deficiencies of trace elements are unusual. However, they may occur on rare occasions if the diet is poor or very limited for a long period of time.

Fat-soluble vitamins		
Name	**Function**	**Dietary sources**
A	For cell development and healthy skin and eyes	Meat, offal, dairy produce, spreading fats, fish oils
D	Controlling calcium balance and bone development	Margarines and fat spreads, cereals, oily fish (in health, also made by the action of sunlight on skin)
E	Antioxidant, protects cells	Spreading fats, meat, fish, eggs, vegetable oils
K	Helps with blood clotting	Green leafy vegetables

The table below gives a summary of some minerals; see page 37 for trace elements.

Many of the minerals, including sodium, potassium and phosphorous, are removed through the kidneys. If the function of your kidneys is

Minerals		
Name/Symbol	**Function**	**Dietary sources**
Sodium (Na)	Essential part of the blood and other body fluids	Table salt, convenience foods, ready meals, fast food
Potassium (K)	Needed for normal muscle and nerve function	Meat, vegetables, fruit, potatoes
Iron (Fe)	Needed to make red blood cells	Red meat, dark green leafy vegetables
Calcium (Ca)	Essential for healthy teeth and bones	Dairy, cheese, milk, yoghurt
Phosphorus (P)	Needed for bones and energy production	Dairy, cheese, milk, yoghurt, offal, shellfish

reduced, your body can lose its ability to remove these minerals as efficiently and they can potentially build up and cause problems (see Chapters 5, 6 and 7).

Iron

Iron helps to make red blood cells, which carry oxygen around the body. A reduced level of red blood cells below the normal level is known as anaemia. In healthy people, anaemia can be caused by not eating enough food containing iron, and is often treated by taking more iron in the diet, or with iron supplements. Anaemia is common in people with kidney failure, but this is primarily because of low levels of a substance called erythropoietin. Erythropoietin is produced by healthy kidneys and normally helps to make red blood cells. If extra iron is needed, this is given as iron tablets or via a drip directly into the blood vessels. It is important to make sure you eat a well balanced diet rather than focusing overly on eating any particular iron-rich foods. This is because some iron-rich foods, such as red meat, should still be eaten in moderation and because following healthy eating advice, such as including fruit and vegetables with meals, will aid the absorption of iron. Avoid drinking tea with your meals as this reduces your body's ability to take in iron from the meal.

Calcium

This mineral is important for the development of bones and teeth. If you are in good health, vitamin D will help your body use the calcium you eat.

Trace elements		
Name/Symbol	**Function**	**Dietary sources**
Zinc (Zn)	Bone health, reproduction and digestion	Meat and pulses
Selenium (Se)	Functions as an antioxidant, protects cells	Meat, fish and cereal grains
Chromium (Cr)	Helps with insulin activity and energy production	Meat, wholegrains, nuts and pulses
Manganese (Mn)	For healthy bones and other functions	Vegetables and tea

However, kidney disease can lead to low levels of vitamin D because of the role of healthy kidneys in forming usable vitamin D in the body. This means your body will find it more difficult to absorb and use calcium. This may result in low blood calcium levels. You may be prescribed a special vitamin D supplement especially suitable for people with CKD. This will help keep your calcium levels normal.

Sodium, potassium and phosphorous are also minerals. See the relevant chapters for more information.

SUPPLEMENTS AND 'ALTERNATIVE' MEDICINES

A vast range of 'natural' or 'alternative' tablets, liquids and foods are now available from supermarkets, pharmacies and health food shops. If you do not have kidney disease, many of these will be safe and may even do you some good. But be warned: very little is known about how such medicines and other substances behave in your body, especially if your kidneys are not working properly. Some Chinese herbal medicines, for example, can be poisonous to the kidneys. So it is very important that you are careful about using any products like this, and if you are thinking about starting one make sure you discuss it with your pharmacist or doctor first.

Do remember too that most of these products have only passed through simple food regulations, rather than the proper scientific testing required for all the medicines you might be prescribed.

10
Healthy living

WHAT IS IT?

If you have chronic kidney disease (CKD), healthy living is a vital part of your treatment and a way to start taking back some control over your own health. It involves a combination of healthy eating and keeping active, along with retaining a positive interest in life. Healthy eating means choosing a diet with the right balance of energy, nutrients and fibre to keep you as healthy as possible for as long as possible. This is a positive step – focus on all the foods you **can** eat as opposed to the foods you think you can't.

> ### *Healthy living with CKD: main aims*
>
> - Eat healthily
> - Control your weight
> - Keep active
> - Stay positive
> - Take responsibility for your health.

DO YOU NEED TO FOLLOW A HEALTHY DIET?

Following a healthy diet should be a priority for most people with CKD. This is because:

1. You may have an increased risk of heart disease, and a healthy diet will help to reduce this risk.

2. It will help you eat the correct balance of nutrients of all kinds within your diet.

3. It allows you to take control of your own health – especially important if there other aspects such as your age or family history of disease that you cannot change.

④ You can help to prevent and treat other conditions you might have such as high blood pressure, diabetes, high blood fats, high blood cholesterol level and obesity. This is very important in protecting your kidneys from further damage and improving your health in the long term.

There are exceptions to this. If you lose your appetite or find eating difficult for any other reason, just eating enough becomes your priority – at least until things improve. In this case, it is advisable to speak to your doctor. You can then be referred to a dietitian if necessary.

HEALTHY EATING – STEPS TO SUCCESS

Eat regular meals including breakfast; don't skip meals
This is good advice for everyone, whether you are overweight, under-weight or about right. Pages 42–44 give information to help you work out your ideal weight. Breakfast can provide a significant amount of essential nutrients as well as setting you up for the day. People who skip meals often get hungry between meals or towards the end of the day and end up filling up on fatty, sugary or salty snacks. They may also binge on larger amounts of food than they would otherwise do in the latter part of the day when their hunger finally gets the better of them.

Eat less fat and fewer fatty foods
This will help to control cholesterol, which is important in reducing your risk of heart disease. If you are overweight then eating less fat can help you to lose weight (see Chapter 4).

If you eat fat, choose healthier fats
Eating unsaturated (polyunsaturated or monounsaturated) fats instead of saturated fats can lower your risk of heart disease by reducing your cho-lesterol level. Unsaturated fats come from plant sources, such as olive, rapeseed, sunflower or soya oils and margarine (see Chapter 4).

Eat fish regularly
The omega-3 oil found in oily fish can help to protect you against heart disease. Oily fish include herring, mackerel, salmon, sardines, trout and fresh (not tinned) tuna. These fish are also a rich source of protein. Aim to eat at least two portions (a portion is about 140 g) of fish a week one of which should be oily. You can choose from fresh, frozen or canned (in

spring water, not brine). The Marine Stewardship Council (MCS) can tell you where to buy fish from sustainable sources: see Appendix 2 for the Council's website address.

Eat less sugar and fewer sugary foods

These foods tend to be high in energy (calories) and low in other nutrients, so should be avoided if you are overweight. They can also lead to tooth decay, especially if eaten between meals.

Eat foods rich in fibre

High fibre foods include wholegrain cereals, wholemeal bread and pasta, brown rice, pulses, lentils and fruit and vegetables. They add taste, texture and interest to your meals. Eating fibre-rich food protects you against heart disease and cancer. It also helps you keep your bowels working normally and avoid constipation. Choosing these high fibre foods can help to fill you up in a healthy way as they are bulky and relatively low in calories. They also tend to have a lower glycaemic index which can help to stabilise blood sugar and reduce hunger pangs (see Chapter 2).

Eat more fruit and vegetables

Fruit and vegetables are tasty, provide vitamins, minerals and fibre and can protect you against heart disease and cancer. The general advice is to aim for five portions of fruit and vegetables each day (see Box below).

A fruit or vegetable portion is about 80 g or roughly a 'handful'

- A whole small banana or medium-sized apple

- A slice of melon

- Two plums or similar-sized fruit

- A small handful of grapes, cherries or berries

- A cereal bowl of salad

- Three heaped tablespoons of vegetables (raw, cooked, frozen or tinned).

Don't worry about eating the latest 'superfood' or fashionable fruit or vegetables. All fruits and vegetables have valuable health benefits which differ according to the nutrients they contain. You should aim to eat as wide a range of different types and colours as you can. Eat fresh, frozen or tinned for convenience. The recipes in this book have been chosen to help you take advantage of the wide variety found in your local shops and supermarkets. Those on a low-potassium diet may need to limit the amount and types of fruit and vegetables, and prepare and cook them in a way that lowers their potassium content (see Chapter 6 for more details).

Eat less salt

We are all advised to eat less salt and this is true, too, for most people who have kidney disease. Avoid adding salt to food and in cooking, as well as keeping clear of salty foods such as processed meat, salted biscuits and bottled sauces. Chapter 5 includes more information on cutting down on salt. All the recipes in this book have been chosen to show you this in practice.

Drink alcohol in moderation only

Unless your doctor advises you to avoid alcohol altogether, you should be able to include alcohol in moderate amounts if you wish. As a general guide, it is advisable to limit yourself to a maximum of 21 units per week for men (no more than 4 units in one day) and 14 units per week for women (no more than 3 units in one day). A unit is equal to half a pint of standard strength beer, a single pub measure of spirits or a small glass of wine. Be aware that drinks you pour yourself are usually larger than standard pub measures. Alcoholic drinks can also be high in calories so cutting down can help with weight loss. You may be advised to limit certain alcoholic (and non-alcoholic) drinks if your blood potassium level is high.

MAINTAINING A HEALTHY WEIGHT

A healthy weight is usually taken to mean the weight at which you have neither too much nor too little body fat. One way to estimate your healthy weight is to calculate your body mass index or BMI which compares your weight with your height (see the chart, overleaf). A BMI of between 20 and 25 is generally recommended as healthy so there will be a range of weights considered to be healthy for your particular height. A BMI of 26–30 is overweight, whereas a BMI over 30 indicates obesity.

$$\text{Body mass index} = \frac{\text{weight (kg)}}{\text{height (m)} \times \text{height (m)}}$$

Example: Agatha is 1.66 m tall and weighs 78 kg

$$\text{BMI} = \frac{78}{1.66 \times 1.66} = 28$$

So Agatha is overweight. A healthy weight range for this height would be 55–69 kg

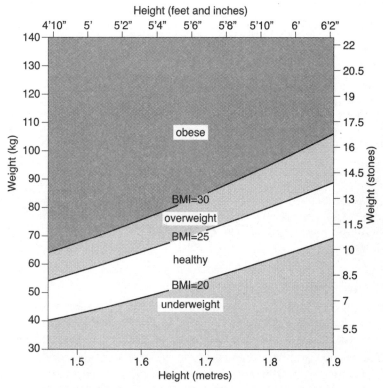

Use the chart or do the calculation above to find out your BMI.

Your BMI score:
below 20: underweight
20–25: ideal/healthy
25–30: overweight
30+: seriously overweight (obese)

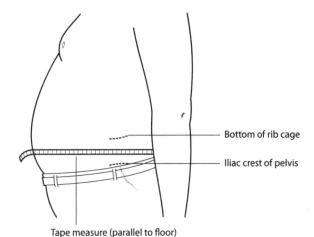

Bottom of rib cage

Iliac crest of pelvis

Tape measure (parallel to floor)

Measuring waist circumference

Waist measurement and health outlook		
	Increased risk to health	*Even greater risk to health*
Men	More than 94 cm (37 in)	More than 102 cm (40 in)
Women	More than 80 cm (32 in)	More than 88 cm (35 in)

*In Asian adults these values differ as follows: 90 cm (35 in) or more in a man, 80 cm (32 in) in a woman would be associated with a greater risk to health. If you are in any doubt about your personal risk, speak to your doctor.

Waist circumference

Measuring your waist (as shown in the diagram) is an easy way to find out whether the fat on your body is stored in places that put your health at greater risk. Individuals who hold most of their fat in and around their abdomen (apple shaped) have a greater risk of developing conditions such as heart disease and diabetes. Whereas people who carry most their fat around their hips (pear shaped) are linked to a lower risk of developing these diseases.

Weight changes with kidney disease

If you have kidney disease, you may retain water in your body which makes your ankles swell. The weight of this water will also mean that you appear to weigh more than you normally do. If you suffer from water retention ask your doctor to help you calculate your BMI with your true weight, which does not include this extra water.

Aim for a healthy weight

If you need to lose weight, the best way to start is to follow the healthy eating guidelines (see pages 40–42). Make sure you are aiming for a realistic and healthy weight while increasing your activity levels as much as you can safely. Some people find that group weight-loss classes or meetings are helpful. Before joining up you will need to make them aware of your medical condition and it is wise to check that their dietary advice is in line with the recommended healthy eating guidelines. Your doctor, nurse or dietitian will always be happy to discuss a suitable approach to weight loss with you and answer any questions you might have.

On the other hand, you may be underweight or have a small appetite and find yourself losing weight without meaning to. In this case you should see your doctor, who may refer you to a dietitian to work out a treatment plan. You will probably be advised to eat more regularly, include snacks between meals and eat more high-energy (calorie) foods.

Weight control and fad diets

'I've found a great diet to help me lose weight – should I use it?'

Fad diets can be very tempting. They usually offer 'quick and easy' ways to lose weight, but weight loss should not be quick. Unfortunately, there is no magic solution to losing weight. If any product sounds too good to be true, it probably is – and it's just the same with weight-loss diets.

If you thinking about trying a weight-loss diet, you need to be careful, particularly if you have kidney disease. If any of the following points apply to the diet you are considering, then don't use it:

- Does it offer a 'miracle' cure or quick fix?

- Does it promote a limited number of particular foods such as cabbage, pineapple, grapefruit etc?

- Does it encourage you to eat an unbalanced diet which does not follow healthy eating guidelines, such as the high-protein, low-carbohydrate diets?

- Would it cost you a lot of money?

- Are there particular tablets, drinks or medication that you have to buy and which are only available from the individual or company promoting the diet?

'Quick fixes' rarely work, and if someone has additional health problems such as kidney disease they may cause real damage. You need to aim for permanent changes to both your diet and your weight. If you don't, your health might suffer and you will find yourself gaining back the weight you have lost.

EXERCISE AND ACTIVITY

Exercise is an essential part of 'healthy living'. Whether you are underweight, overweight or somewhere in between, it is important for you to think about the type and amount of exercise you do.

Exercise will help you build and maintain muscle. If you are overweight, being more active will help you to lose fat, gain muscle and reach and maintain a healthy weight.

Exercise can also help if you have trouble sleeping, feel anxious or depressed, and can lead to increased self-confidence, independence and a

---

If you are not exercising you are missing out!

Exercise can help to:

- ✔ Reduce overweight
- ✔ Improve muscle size and strength
- ✔ Prevent falls
- ✔ Reduce insomnia and improve sleep patterns
- ✔ Reduce anxiety and depression
- ✔ Improve overall energy levels
- ✔ Increase self-confidence
- ✔ Improve bone strength
- ✔ Help to control diabetes and high blood pressure
- ✔ Help to control blood fats and sugars
- ✔ Help with treatment for anaemia
- ✔ Improve your social life

feeling of well-being. Exercise can improve bone strength, protect against osteoporosis and help with other conditions common in people with kidney disease, including raised blood pressure, diabetes and high cholesterol.

In fact, if you are not doing any form of exercise, you are missing out on a great benefit. It doesn't have to be expensive, difficult or embarrassing. Simple lifestyle changes such as walking further and more often are cheap, easily available, and can prevent and treat many of the conditions from which you may suffer, now or in the future. Studies have shown that those people who do little or no exercise have the most to gain from increasing their daily activity levels.

What can you do?

Anything that makes you more active will provide you with exercise. Some ideas that involve you increasing your activity are:

- Getting up to change channels on the TV instead of using the remote control;

- Walking to the shops instead of driving;

- Collecting your morning paper instead of having it delivered;

- Getting off the bus one or two stops earlier and walking the rest of the way;

- Doing some housework or gardening;

- Using the stairs instead of a lift or escalator;

- Walking the dog, or offering to walk someone else's;

- Doing 'chair exercises' (exercising while seated);

- Playing active games or sport with your own (or borrowed) children, grandchildren, godchildren, nephews or nieces.

You could also take up an active pastime or learn a new skill such as pilates, yoga, cycling, line dancing, gardening or aqua-aerobics. This can be a great for your social life as well as your waistline.

Becoming more active

Start by deciding what you would like to do and making a real commitment to doing it. Whatever you choose to do, it will help if it is something you enjoy. Start off gently and build up gradually – your aim is to try to make your body work a little harder, perhaps from a brisk walk rather than a stroll. Try walking in the park, the countryside or even just around the block. As a general rule you shouldn't do anything that makes you too out of breath to talk and – obviously – you should avoid doing anything that hurts. Although you shouldn't worry if you haven't done any exercise for a long time, it is always a good idea to check with your GP or clinic doctor before starting any new form of exercise. Your doctor will also be able to advise you about suitable ways to increase your activity levels and direct you to information on local facilities. You could also visit your local community or leisure centre, library or place of worship, look on your local council's website or ask your friends or family for more ideas on activities you might enjoy.

How much should I be doing?

We should all aim to be doing 30 minutes of exercise five times a week. This should be done at a moderate intensity so that your heart rate is faster than normal and you feel warm, but you should still have enough breath to talk. You can break this down into three 10-minute sessions or two 15-minute sessions if you prefer.

Barriers	Solutions
I don't have time to exercise.	Exercise can be built into your daily routine. Every little bit helps. Start with 10 minutes and gradually build up.
I am too tired after work.	Plan to do something active before work or during the day.
I cannot afford to join a gym.	There are many types of exercise that you can do for free such as walking, using tins for weights.
It's boring.	Find something you enjoy doing and take friends along, e.g. walking, salsa dancing.
I am too old.	You can be active at any age.

11
Diabetes

Over two million people in the UK have diabetes, a condition which affects the control of sugar in the blood. This can result in high blood sugar levels which can damage the kidneys as well as other parts of the body such as the eyes. Diabetes is a common condition in people with chronic kidney disease (CKD) and often, but not always, a cause of the kidney damage. This means that many people who are diagnosed with CKD are already trying to keep to the dietary recommendations for diabetes. If you are one of them, you may be worried that you will have to cope with lots of additional or conflicting dietary advice for your CKD. Therefore, it may be helpful to know that the suggested diets for both CKD and diabetes are really very similar. This is because the shared main aim for the diet is to help to prevent and treat heart disease through healthy, balanced eating (see Box below). Control of body weight and blood pressure are two further shared goals. So the good news is that making these basic changes to your diet is worth doing – you can really improve your overall health as well as tackling the CKD.

Healthy living with diabetes

- Eat regular meals

- Have wholegrain starchy foods at each meal

- Eat more fruit and vegetables

- Reduce fat and fatty foods

- Reduce salt

- Reduce sugar and sugary foods

- Limit alcohol

- Keep to a healthy body weight

- Increase daily activity levels.

The one main area that people with diabetes sometimes find confusing is the advice on fruit and vegetables. They are generally encouraged to have 'plenty' – at least five 80 g portions daily. Five portions of fruit and vegetables a day are fine for most people with diabetes and CKD. The exception is those with high blood potassium levels who may need to limit their fruit and vegetables (see Chapter 6). This doesn't mean that fruit and vegetables are not beneficial, just that they cannot be eaten as freely because of their potassium content. It is also important to note that potassium is not in itself harmful; usually it is considered to be positively beneficial. It only needs to be limited by those whose kidneys are not working well enough to control their blood potassium levels.

GLYCAEMIC INDEX

Starchy carbohydrate foods are converted into sugar in the body. This means that they will increase your blood sugar level. This happens at different rates, depending on the type and form of the food. The glycaemic index (GI) of a carbohydrate food is the rate at which the food is digested to release the sugar (glucose) it contains into the blood. Foods which have a lower glycaemic index are thought to be most beneficial for people with diabetes as the rise in blood sugar is slower and easier to control (Chapter 2 has more information about this).

12
Different tastes and socialising

Being told that you have chronic kidney disease (CKD) doesn't have to mean you should stop going out and socialising, eating food you like, exploring different tastes and sharing in special occasions. By taking a few sensible precautions, you can continue to enjoy your chosen lifestyle to a much greater degree than you may have feared.

EATING OUT

The amount of attention you pay to your diet when you are not at home really depends on how often you eat out. An occasional meal is unlikely to make much difference to your overall diet. But if you eat out at least once a week, you may need to choose your menu with a bit more care. Just as at home, your choices will depend on your own particular tastes, medical condition, blood results and lifestyle.

The main exception to this is if you need to follow a low-potassium diet. You will always need to be 'potassium aware' whether it is a one-off meal, or a regular event. This is because even short-term rises in potassium levels in the body can be harmful.

Unless your doctor has advised you otherwise, it is fine to include alcohol with meals and other social occasions, but drink it in moderation. Alcoholic drinks are quite high in calories, and some types also contain a fair amount of potassium. Alcohol can also interfere with control of diabetes if you have it. Therefore, remember to ask for information about alcohol when you are seeing your doctor or dietitian. It can also weaken your efforts to resist tempting extras – would you really have that extra bag of crisps or the greasy takeaway if you were stone-cold sober?

Stay away from nibbles!
It will really help to keep well away from salty nibbles and snacks, such as crisps, nuts, Bombay mix, pastries, samosas, fried fish cakes, potato shapes etc. These are often high in fat and calories and it's hard to keep track of exactly what you have eaten. They may also make you thirsty and cause

you to drink more sugary or alcoholic drinks. But for many of us, the worst thing about nibbles is that once you start you can't stop!

- **Tip:** Try a longer drink! Add a sugar-free or low-calorie mixer to your alcohol to make it go further:
- Shandy – sugar-free lemonade with lager
- Spritzer – sparkling water with white or rosé wine
- Gin and slimline tonic
- Vodka with low-sugar cranberry juice

Thinking ahead

Preparing yourself and the people who are cooking for you can make all the difference. For example:

- If you are going to a restaurant, try to contact the manager in advance. Ask about the choice of food, and discuss any special arrangements that might be needed.

- If you have been invited to someone else's home, you will make meal planning much easier for your hosts if you phone ahead to discuss what you can and can't eat.

- If you know that you might be eating a less suitable food for dinner at a friend's house, you might just decide that you will be more careful during the day to compensate. For example, you could avoid that tempting sausage sandwich for breakfast to allow for the extra calories/fat/salt later on.

- A few simple changes to the way food is prepared and served can make a meal much easier for you to eat. Butter, sauces, gravy and salad dressings can be served separately or left out altogether; a high-potassium vegetable or fruit may be changed for a low-potassium alternative; garnishes can be omitted.

FOODS FROM AROUND THE WORLD

Our multicultural society offers a wealth of eating experiences both at home and when eating out. Talking to your health adviser about the sort of diet you and your family like to eat can be very helpful. They may be

DOs and DON'Ts for eating out

DO try to plan ahead – you may be able to adjust your diet before or after the meal out to allow for any foods and drinks that you would not normally have.

DO consider how often you eat out when deciding how flexible to be with your diet.

DO try to choose suitable foods when you are out. If you run into difficulties choose only a small amount of the unfamiliar food.

DO remember to allow for alcoholic or non-alcoholic drinks as part of any social occasion or a meal out, especially if you are on a reduced-calorie, low-potassium or fluid-restricted diet.

DO ask your host or waiter to serve the food appropriately. For example, many sauces, dressings, garnishes and other extras can often be served separately or left out altogether.

DON'T be afraid to ask the restaurant, café or takeaway to change a dish to suit your requirements. It's often worth telephoning ahead to check that they will have something that you are happy to eat.

DON'T forget to ask your dietitian for advice on eating meals out and at special occasions. Dietitians will be happy to provide information (both for you and for your relatives and friends) that is geared to your own particular diet and needs.

unfamiliar with your particular diet, but are likely to be keen to learn from you. If you see a dietitian, he or she will work together with you to ensure that any dietary changes don't have to stop you from eating your traditional or family foods.

Here are a few general tips to consider when choosing some of your favourite meals.

Chinese and Thai

- Food from China and the Far East can be very salty. Avoid adding salt or salty sauces such as soy sauce or fish sauce. Ask for food without added MSG (monosodium glutamate), another source of sodium. Reduced-salt soy sauce is available but still needs to be used sparingly.

- Plain boiled or steamed rice or noodles are suitable accompaniments to any meal. Fried noodles and rice are higher in fat and energy but if you include them try to make sure they are cooked in a 'healthy oil' such as sunflower, soya or rapeseed oils (see Chapter 10).

- Many typical flavourings (ginger, garlic, allspice, lemongrass) can be enjoyed freely for a delicious taste on a low-salt diet.

- If you choose a dish which comes with plenty of sauce, such as a Thai curry, try to leave much of the sauce behind in the serving dish. This will cut down on the amount of salt and fat (and potassium) that you eat.

- Stir-fries can be a convenient option to retain more of the taste and nutrients in your meal – especially if cooked at home with a minimal amount of fat. They are a good way to include plenty of vegetables in your meal. If you are on a low-potassium diet, count them within your vegetable allowance or as advised.

Italian and Mediterranean

- As a starchy carbohydrate, pasta is a good basis to a meal and its low glycaemic index will keep you fuller for longer. Avoid those rich creamy or cheesy sauces – add plenty of vegetables instead.

- Olive oil is a monounsaturated fat and an essential part of the 'Mediterranean' healthy approach to eating. However, it is just as high in calories as any other fat.

- A low-salt dressing for fish, meat and vegetables can be made from balsamic vinegar or lemon juice, olive oil and black pepper. You can limit the oil or leave it out altogether if you are trying to lose weight.

- Bread is tasty and convenient; Italy and other Mediterranean countries have a wide range of breads to choose from. Try ciabatta, pitta bread or breadsticks as an accompaniment or starter. However, watch out for the saltier breads, such as foccacia and those with added ingredients such as olives or even salt crystals.

- Wherever possible avoid adding extra parmesan or other hard cheeses to dishes, as they are high in salt and saturated fat. Soft cheeses such as ricotta, mascarpone and cream cheese are lower in salt and you should be able to find low-fat versions or alternatives to use at home.

- Pizza is another favourite, but often salty and high in fat with all that cheese on top. Avoid 'stuffed-crust' or similar American-style pizzas and salty ingredients such as anchovies, olives, cured meats. Ask for less cheese and extra vegetables instead. Try our recipe for homemade pizza or add your own (healthy) toppings to a bought base for a quick meal at home.

Indian/Indian subcontinent

- Use the minimum of oil to prepare curries and other dishes at home. Trim all fat from meat and remove skin from poultry before using. You do not want to be able to see a layer of oil on the finished dish.

- When eating out, try to leave some of the sauce in the serving dish and just eat the meat, fish or vegetables – this will cut down on the salt and fat you eat. You can achieve the same effect at home by serving food with a slotted spoon.

- Try to avoid choosing dishes made with fattier ingredients such as creamed coconut or cream. At home replace with lower-fat alternatives such as reduced-fat coconut milk, yoghurt or fromage frais.

- Boiled rice is a good accompaniment to your meal. At home cook without adding salt but you can try adding lemon rind, cinnamon stick, cloves, turmeric or saffron to the cooking water for extra flavour.

- When cooking at home, keep to unsaturated 'healthy' oils such as rapeseed (often sold as 'vegetable' oil), corn, sunflower oils instead of butter or ghee. Still use as little as possible if you are watching your weight as all oils and fats are high in calories.

- Avoid deep-fried snacks and starters. Try baked or grilled snacks instead. Uncooked popadum disks can be cooked in the microwave instead of frying.

- There is a great choice of fruit and vegetables to sample. If you are on a potassium restriction your dietitian can help you include them safely.

- Keep your salt intake down by avoiding salty pickles, chutneys and ready made 'curry' sauces – try using more naturally low-salt flavours such as fresh herbs, fresh and dried chillis, garlic, ginger, lemon, limes and traditional spices.

African / Caribbean

- Stews and 'soups' are a traditional way to serve meat or fish with vegetables in one dish. Using a slotted spoon to dish up a portion of stew allows the liquid to drain away and reduces the fat, salt (and potassium) content of the meal.

- A wide range of starchy staples such as plain rotis, rice, ground rice, and couscous make a healthy basis to any meal. Sweet potato and especially yams and cassava are low GI choices. If you are on a low-potassium diet, try to boil vegetables, potatoes and other starchy staples, before eating or adding them to stews and similar dishes.

- To cut down on your sodium (salt) intake, try to avoid dishes containing salted meats and fish. Fresh meat and fish are good alternatives. Trim away meat fat and remove poultry skin before using. If you are preparing salted meat or fish at home, soak and rinse thoroughly in plenty of water to wash away some of the salt.

- A wide range of flavourings can be enjoyed including fresh and dried thyme, coriander and other herbs, garlic, chilli, allspice and other spices.

- Limit nuts, including coconut and peanuts, if you are on a low-calorie, low-phosphate or low-potassium diet. Choose reduced-fat coconut milk instead of the standard version.

CELEBRATIONS AND SPECIAL OCCASIONS

Family, national and religious holidays and celebrations can have a great influence on how we eat. From birthdays and bank holidays, to Chanukah, Eid and Diwali, many occasions have special foods and meals associated with them. Christmas, in particular, is associated with a vast range of seasonal foods that are available for several weeks of the year and will probably affect your diet whether or not Christmas is part of your own family traditions.

Hints and tips for celebrations

- Roast meats such as turkey, pork, beef or lamb are a good choice eaten hot or cold. Instead of using salt, try cooking with lemon, garlic, black pepper, spices or fresh herbs such as rosemary to add flavour.

- Gravy and bottled sauces can be very high in salt and/ or fat. Fortunately cranberry sauce, mint sauce, and homemade mustard (make up the powder with water or vinegar) are popular exceptions to this rule. A big portion of vegetables will keep things moist and tasty without adding lots of gravy.

- Many special occasion foods tend to be high in potassium, especially around Christmas time. These include some of the vegetables such as parsnips, roast potatoes, yams and Brussels sprouts as well as dried fruit, crisps, nuts, chocolates, Indian sweetmeats and fried snacks, fruit juices and fortified wines. If you are on a potassium restriction, you will need to eat them sparingly to keep your potassium levels under control. Ask your dietitian for advice on enjoying seasonal foods without harming your health.

- Many savoury nibbles, such as crisps, pakora, nuts and Bombay mix are high in salt. Try lower salt alternatives such as unsalted crackers, crisps, tortilla chips, fried/baked vegetable or apple crisps. Have a few walnuts, pecans (buy them unshelled and you tend to eat less) and roasted chestnuts, or try fresh fruit.

- Both sweet and savoury nibbles can be very high in fat and calories

– and once you start it's difficult to stop! Try to avoid them or decide on a limit, especially around Christmas or other festive periods where they are constantly available.

- Dried fruit (figs, currants, dates, prunes etc.) are a high-fibre, low-fat sweet treat if you do not need to restrict your potassium intake. Other special occasion fruit – such as pineapple, strawberries, melon, cherries and grapes – can make healthy sweet desserts and snacks. Raw vegetables (carrots, red pepper, cauliflower etc.) are good for dipping – try low-fat salsas or yoghurt dips, homemade houmous or vegetable dips instead of the creamy or cheesy kind (see recipe section).

13
Practical hints

We have talked about the theory of eating with chronic kidney disease (CKD); now it is time to turn it all into practice. This section of the book gives you some basic checklists: conversion charts, hints on using herbs and spices, advice on labelling and tips on food hygiene.

CONVERSION CHARTS

All the conversions below are approximate. In all our recipes, spoon measurements are level unless otherwise stated.

Weights		Volume	
Metric	*Imperial*	*Metric*	*Imperial*
7 g	¼ oz	5 ml	1 teaspoon
15 g	½ oz	15 ml	1 tablespoon
20 g	¾ oz	30 ml	2 tablespoons
25 g	1 oz	100 ml	3½ fl oz
40 g	1½ oz	125 ml	4 fl oz
50 g	2 oz	150 ml	¼ pint
75 g	3 oz	175 ml	6 fl oz
125 g	4 oz	200 ml	7 fl oz
150 g	5 oz	225 ml	8 fl oz
175 g	6 oz	250 ml	9 fl oz
200 g	7 oz	300 ml	½ pint
250 g	8 oz	350 ml	12 fl oz
275 g	9 oz	400 ml	14 fl oz
300 g	10 oz	450 ml	¾ pint
325 g	11 oz	500 ml	18 fl oz
375 g	12 oz	600 ml	1 pint
400 g	13 oz	700 ml	1¼ pints
425 g	14 oz	900 ml	1½ pints
450 g	15 oz	1 litre	1¾ pints
500 g	17½ oz	2 litres	3½ pints
1 kg	2 lb 3 oz	2.75 litres	5 pints

Measurements

Metric	Imperial
5 mm	¼ inch
1 cm	½ inch
2 cm	1 inch
5 cm	2 inches
7 cm	3 inches
10 cm	4 inches
12 cm	5 inches
15 cm	6 inches
18 cm	7 inches
20 cm	8 inches
23 cm	9 inches
25 cm	10 inches
28 cm	11 inches
30 cm	12 inches

Oven temperatures

(For fan ovens, adjust the cooking temperature in accordance with the manufacturer's instructions)

Celsius	Fahrenheit	Gas Mark	Description
110°C	225°F	¼	cool
120°C	250°F	½	cool
140°C	275°F	1	very low
150°C	300°F	2	very low
160°C	325°F	3	low
180°C	350°F	4	moderate
190°C	375°F	5	moderate
200°C	400°F	6	mod hot
220°C	425°F	7	hot
230°C	450°F	8	hot
240°C	475°F	9	very hot

FLAVOURING WITH HERBS AND SPICES

You can use herbs and spices to help to reduce your salt intake without losing out on flavour. In our recipes we have tried to cut out or minimise the addition of salt as far as possible. Below is a list of some other suggestions you may also wish to try. As a rule of thumb, dried herbs and spices are best added into 'moist' foods such as soups, stews and sauces during cooking. Fresh herbs are widely available and add flavour to almost any dish. Your local Asian, Mediterranean or other speciality stores often have the best deals on fresh herbs and will be able to advise on their use. Some of the more delicate varieties such as coriander and basil are best added just before serving. Others, such as rosemary and thyme, release their flavour during cooking.

Many herbs are easy to grow, in the garden or on a window sill, and plants or seeds are readily available. Frozen herbs can be bought or made easily at home. Chop up the herbs and cover with a little water in an ice cube tray, then freeze. They will then be in convenient portion sizes for later use.

Herbs	
Basil	**Fresh** – Add a chopped leaf or two to salad, or to pasta, stews and other hot dishes before serving. **Dried** – Add a pinch into stews or sprinkled on beef before roasting.
Bay leaf	Use a couple of dried leaves in stocks and stews or when boiling potatoes.
Chives	Chop a few fresh chives and add to a potato salad, cottage cheese, or serve with chicken or fish.
Mint	Use a fresh sprig with vegetables or on a little lamb before grilling.
Parsley	More than just a garnish . . . great with chicken, fish and vegetables.
Sage	Add fresh or dried sage to home-made stuffings for pork or poultry; also good with roast vegetables or potatoes.
Tarragon	A little fresh or dried tarragon goes well with chicken or fish; fresh tarragon is also tasty on a salad.
Thyme	Use in stews, or in home-made stuffing for poultry and game.
Mixed herbs	Try a pinch of dry or fresh, for stuffings, stews, omelettes, pizza.

BUYING INGREDIENTS OR READY-MADE FOODS: READING THE LABELS

There are two main ways supermarkets and food manufacturers are trying to help us to identify foods which are 'healthier' – this is usually understood to be foods which are lower in fat, saturated fat, sugar and salt.

'Traffic Light System'

This is a system launched by the Food Standards Agency to help us identify at a glance if the food is high, medium or low in fat, saturated fat, sugar and salt. It has been adopted by many of the supermarkets, food stores, food manufacturers and some food outlets. There are several versions in use but all use the same coding system:

- **Red** The food is high in something that we should be trying to cut down on. These foods should be eaten in smaller amounts only occasionally.

- **Amber** This food is neither high nor low in the nutrient. These foods can be taken occasionally, but try to keep to more green lights.

- **Green** The more green lights, the healthier the food. This is because it is low in fat, saturated fat, salt or sugar. Try to keep to more of these foods.

Many foods will have a mixture of traffic lights. Aim to choose foods with more amber and green lights and fewer red lights. (For more information see the website www.eatwell.gov.uk).

GDA – Guideline daily amounts

Guideline daily amounts (GDA) are a guide to how many calories, how much fat, saturated fat, sugar and salt a typical adult should be eating each day. If you are more active, your GDA will be higher, and if you are less active your GDA will be lower.

Images are used to show the amount of calories, fat, saturated fat, sugar and salt in each serving of the food. This is also shown as a percentage of the GDA.

Foods which contain a high percentage of your GDA (for calories, fats, sugar or salt) should be taken only occasionally and in small amounts. Foods with a lower percentage of your GDA will tend to be the healthier options. GDA are sometimes used in combination with the traffic light system. One disadvantage of using GDA is that few of us will need quite the same as the 'typical' adult identified by this system.

Chicken salad – example of GDA	
Each pack contains:	
260 kcal	13% GDA
4.8 g fat	7% GDA
1.1 g salt	19% GDA

Ingredients
Labels on most packed foods must list all the ingredients. The ingredients are listed in descending order of weight at the time of their use in the preparation of the food.

Nutritional content
This must be given per 100 g but many labels also have information per serving. Where per serving information is given, the weight or portion size has to be stated, as in the example of a ready-made chicken curry, pictured overleaf.

Comparing meals and foods
When comparing different meals or foods, you need to look at the amount of nutrient there is per 100 g. To get an idea whether your chosen meal has a lot or a little of a particular nutrient, use the 'ready reckoner' below as a guide. If you are comparing ingredients, you may also want to look at how much of that ingredient there is in the final cooked meal.

READY RECKONER (per 100 g of food)	
A lot	**A little**
10.0 g sugars	2.0 g sugars
20.0 g fat	3.0 g fat
5.0 g saturates	1.0 g saturates
3.0 g fibre	0.5 g fibre
0.5 g sodium	0.1 g sodium

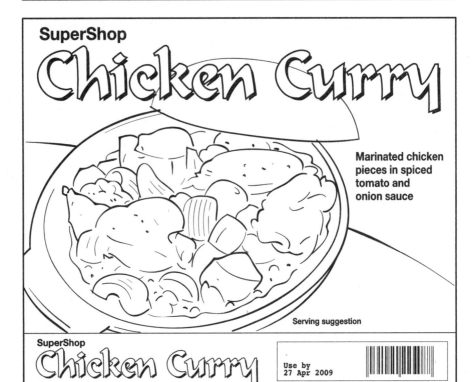

SuperShop

Chicken Curry

Marinated chicken pieces in spiced tomato and onion sauce

Serving suggestion

SuperShop

Chicken Curry

Use by
27 Apr 2009

Cooking Guidelines

Oven
35 – 40 mins
190°C/375°F

Microwave
650 watt – category B 5½ mins
750 watt – category D 5 mins
850 watt – category E 4½ mins
• For best results microwave heat
• Remove outer packaging
• Pierce lid several times
• Heat on full power
• Stir well before serving

Freezing
• Freeze on day of purchase
• For freezing guidelines refer to
  manufacturer's handbook

Oven from frozen
45 – 50 mins
190°C/375°F
• Follow oven instructions above,
  adjusting heating time to
  45–50 mins.

Storage
• Keep refrigerated
• Use by: see side of packet

SuperShop

Chicken Curry

Marinated chicken pieces in spiced tomato and onion sauce

Nutrition

Typical Compos-ition	A 350g serving provides	A 100g serving provides
Energy	1460kj	417kj
	350kcal	100kcal
Protein	32.6g	9.3g
Carbohydrate	12.3g	3.5g
of which sugars	9.5g	2.7g
Fat	32.9g	9.4g
Fibre	5.3g	1.5g
Sodium	2.1g	0.6g

350g

Produced in the United Kingdom for
SuperShop Stores

Ingredients

Marinated chicken (51%)
Tomato (19%)
Onion (7%)
Vegetable Oil (5.1%)
Tomato Purée
Garlic Purée
Ginger Purée
Coriander
Chicken Stock
Ground Coriander
Onion Purée
Ground Cumin
Minced Green Chillies
Chicken Fat
Salt

Every care has been made to remove bones,
but some may still remain

Going back to the chicken curry example, the label indicates that it contains a moderate amount of fat (9.4 g per 100 g of product), making it a reasonably acceptable choice. But it does contain quite a high level of salt (0.6 g sodium per 100 g of product).

Labelling claims

Food labels cannot just say anything they would like to as labelling is strictly governed by law. A food cannot claim to be 'reduced calorie' unless it is much lower in calories than the usual version. Nevertheless, claims made on packaging need to be interpreted with care. This is because, with the exception of butters, margarines and other spreadable fats, the law states no legal definitions for quantities but states the claim should not be misleading and gives several recommendations.

It is useful to understand what these recommendations are to be able to compare similar foods and assess the most suitable food choice for you and your dietary goals.

'Reduced fat'

When a food has a reduction claim in a nutrient (such as 'reduced fat') it is important to remember what the standard product is like to make a true assessment of the benefit of this claim. For example, we all know that pork pies are a very high-fat food. Legally, if the manufacturers reduced the fat content in the recipe by 25%, they could claim the product was 'Reduced Fat'. However, while the reduced fat option might be better than the standard product, it would still be a significant source of fat.

'Low fat'

In addition, 'low' or 'lower' in fat does not mean that the product is also low in sugar. It may even have more sugar than the original standard product. Similarly 'low in sugar' makes no claim about the fat content. There is no guarantee either that low-fat and low-sugar products are lower in calories. Often they are as high – or almost as high – in calories as the full-fat or full-sugar product.

'No added'

Some products carry the claim 'no added sugar (or salt)'. Again this term means that that no sugar (or salt) has been added in the manufacturing process; it does not always mean it is actually low in these nutrients. For example, we know from an average supermarket label of pure, unsweetened orange juice that a typical sugar content of 10.5 g per

100 ml means that it can still be a rich source of sugar if too much is consumed.

Potassium and phosphate

Potassium and phosphate are rarely included in the nutritional information in the UK as it relatively rare for these nutrients to be restricted in the diet. Therefore, if you have been advised to follow a low-potassium or phosphate diet you will have to look instead at the main ingredients used. In many cases, it is also helpful to think about how the dish or food is likely to have been cooked and prepared. You might be able to compare it with a similar dish that you make at home.

Going back to the Chicken Curry label on page 64:

- Tomatoes come second in the descending order of ingredients, and make up 19% of the weight of ingredients used. As tomatoes are relatively high in potassium, this dish is also likely to be high in potassium. If you have been asked to be careful with the amount of potassium you eat, it may not necessarily mean you can never choose this dish. But options to consider could be:

- Choose another curry dish that uses less tomato.

- Choose a low-potassium accompaniment such as plain rice or naan.

- Reduce the amount of other foods that are high in potassium to be eaten earlier on that day, or the day after, to 'make room' for this choice.

These strategies can also apply to other nutrients such as fat, salt, sugar and calories. For example, if you are choosing a dish high in any of these, try eating it with appropriate accompaniments such as a salad, boiled vegetables or boiled rice, instead of less suitable choices such as chips, fried rice or salted tinned vegetables.

FOOD HYGIENE

When storing, preparing and cooking food it is always good practice to follow basic principles of food hygiene to help minimise any risk of food infection. These are some general guidelines:

- Take chilled and frozen food home quickly, then put it in your fridge or freezer promptly. Do not refreeze thawed food.

- Prepare and store raw and cooked food separately – keep raw meat and fish at the bottom of your fridge.

- Keep the coldest part of your fridge at 0–5°C. Consider buying a fridge thermometer if you don't already have one.

- Check 'use by' dates, and use food within the recommended period.

- Keep pets away from food and worktops.

- Wash your hands thoroughly before preparing food or eating.

- Wash worktops and utensils between preparing raw and cooked food.

- Do not eat foods containing uncooked eggs. Keep your eggs in the fridge.

- Cook your food well. Make sure you follow any instructions on the pack and if you reheat, ensure the food is piping hot. Do not reheat food more than once.

- Keep hot foods HOT and cold foods COLD; do not just leave them standing around at room temperature.

MEAL PLANNING

Good meal planning enables you to get the best possible balance of nutrients in the most enjoyable way. It's about getting the taste, texture, colour and smell of the meal right, as well as making sure that what you eat is good for you. We hope that reading through this book will have given you plenty of ideas about doing just this, but here are a few tips to help you make the most of the recipes. Planning meals for a restricted diet can seem a huge challenge. The recipes in this book have been chosen to show you how the old favourites can work well with a restricted diet and to introduce you to some new flavours, ingredients and ways of cooking. This should help to make your meals and snacks delicious, easy to prepare and fit in with any dietary changes you have been advised to make.

Eating well
The 'eatwell plate' has been produced by the Food Standards Agency to show how much of what we eat should come from each food group. It can give us an idea how to structure each meal, although the overall balance of the diet based on the 'eatwell plate' includes everything we eat during

The eatwell plate

Use the eatwell plate to help you get the balance right. It shows how much of what you eat should come from each food group.

FOOD
STANDARDS
AGENCY

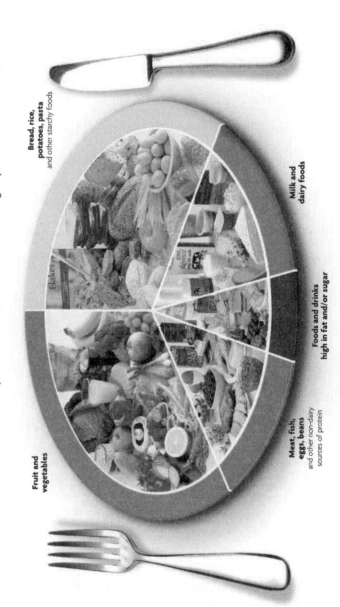

Bread, rice, potatoes, pasta and other starchy foods

Fruit and vegetables

Milk and dairy foods

Meat, fish, eggs, beans and other non-dairy sources of protein

Foods and drinks high in fat and/or sugar

The eatwell plate
Crown copyright 2007, Food Standards Agency

the day, including snacks. Although aimed at the wider community, it is also useful for people with CKD as well those with diabetes, high blood pressure and those who want to control their body weight.

Principles for a well-balanced diet

- **Choose a starchy food for the basis of all your meals** Rice, pasta, noodles, potatoes, yam, bread, breakfast cereals; the list is endless. Some are lower GI or higher in fibre but most can be enjoyed as part of a healthy diet. Add less butter, margarine or oil and you will keep the calories and fat content down. If you need a low-potassium diet, boiling potatoes, yams and other vegetables before eating or cooking further will help to control your potassium intake.

- **Balance your nutrients** If you are eating a food that is high in a restricted nutrient, combine it with a food that is very low in the same nutrient and you may find that the meal is a better fit for your diet. For example, try boiled potatoes and peas with your fried fish instead of chips and baked beans to help keep your salt and fat intake down.

- **Watch out for salt!** Read packets and tins and choose the varieties with less or no added salt, such as tuna in spring water, low-salt baked beans or unsalted breakfast cereals. At home, chuck out your salt pot and add pepper, lemon juice, herbs, spices and all the other salt-free flavours instead. Perhaps you automatically add salt to foods such as pasta, rice or vegetables, so leave it out and you may not even notice. If you make your own bread, try cutting down the salt used in the recipe by a third or more. Experiment with herbs and other flavours instead. There are loads of homemade and bought alternatives to salty sauces.

- **Remember to eat enough fruit and vegetables** Aim for your five (80 g) portions a day unless told otherwise. They can be a great way to add taste, colour, texture and moisture to a meal without extra salt and fluid, as well as providing many essential vitamins, minerals and other essential nutrients. Some fruits and vegetables are high in potassium so people on a low-potassium diet should speak to a dietitian to help them make the best choices. Juices and smoothies can be relatively high in sugar, calories and potassium so limit these if you are concerned about these nutrients.

- **Keep positive** Use the information in this book and the advice from your own dietitian to adjust and adapt your favourite recipes or those in other recipe books. Many of the hints and tips in this book come from people who are following a special diet themselves and have discovered a different way to make their favourite dish taste good without adding salt or another restricted ingredient. Perhaps you may not even make any of the recipes in this book but just pick up some new ideas for making your own meals and snacks taste good. We hope to make it as easy as possible for you to eat food that is both tasty and healthy. Whether reading, cooking or eating, enjoy!

Part 2 – RECIPES

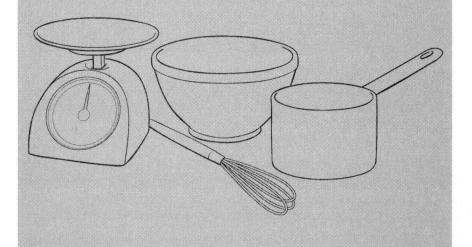

Recipe coding

All our recipes are controlled for salt, fat and saturated fat in order to be suitable for inclusion in a chronic kidney disease (CKD) healthy eating diet. Nutritional analysis of all recipes can be found in Appendix 2 (pages 140–41).

* **Fat** Fat content has been controlled by selecting low-fat ingredients, limiting added fats and avoiding added saturated fat. 'Vegetable oil' refers to rapeseed oil (often labelled as 'vegetable oil'). Otherwise use corn oil, sunflower oil or similar polyunsaturated oil of your choice. Olive oil is also a suitable choice and adds flavour to savoury recipes but may tend to burn at higher temperatures.

* **Low sodium/salt** All dishes have no added salt and have a sodium content of less than 0.3 g per 100 g. If you prefer to use stock instead of water in some recipes, it is advisable to use low-salt stock cubes.

* **Fruit and vegetable portions** The approximate minimum number of portions per serving is indicated by graphic representing apples:

     = one portion

     = half portion

Fruit and vegetable portions are based on 80 g serving or follow government guidelines (see www.eatwell.gov.uk) or manufacturer's labelling.

* **For Diabetes** Suitability as part of a balanced, low-sugar diabetic diet. Only desserts are coded as all savoury dishes would be suitable. Any necessary modifications to the recipe are noted.

SOUPS AND STARTERS

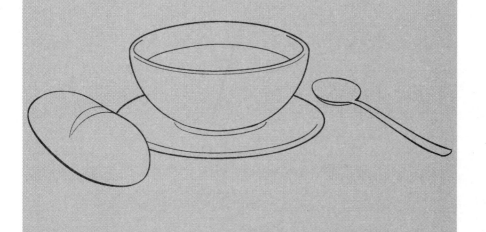

Baked tomatoes

Preparation time:
15 minutes

Cooking time:
20 minutes

Fruit/veg per serving:
🍎

A simple and tasty starter with a great combination of flavours. Eat on its own or with some bread, couscous or perhaps a jacket potato for a more substantial snack.

Ingredients *(serves 2)*
tomatoes • 2 large
garlic • 2 cloves
fresh parsley • 1 bunch
onion • 1 small
black pepper • to taste
wholemeal bread • 2 slices, lightly toasted
olive oil • 2 teaspoons

Slice the tomatoes and place them in a lightly oiled ovenproof dish with the chopped garlic.

Finely chop the garlic, onions and parsley and sprinkle over the tomatoes. Season with black pepper to taste.

To make the breadcrumbs, either crumble the toasted wholemeal bread by hand or use a blender or food processor.

Cover the tomatoes with the breadcrumbs and drizzle over a little olive oil. Bake for about 20 minutes at 180°C or until the breadcrumbs turn a golden brown.

Cook's tip: The tomatoes also make a good accompaniment to a piece of baked fish or roast meat – especially if it can all be cooked at the same time in the oven. No gravy or salty sauces will be needed.

Courgette and carrot soup

Preparation time:
15 minutes

Cooking time:
•40 minutes

Fruit/veg per serving:
🍎🍎🍏

This soup was invented by a gardener with a glut of home-grown courgettes and the flavour is enhanced by an unusual combination of herbs and spices instead of salt. It is a great way to eat your vegetables at any time of year.

Ingredients *(serves 4)*

vegetable oil • 2 tablespoons
onion • 1, finely chopped (200 g)
garlic • 2 cloves, chopped
courgettes • 300 g
carrots • 300 g
powdered cumin • ½ teaspoon
water or low-salt stock • 500 ml
black pepper • to taste
fresh basil leaves • 2 tablespoons, chopped

Heat the oil in a large saucepan and soften the onion and garlic for 3–4 minutes. Take care not to burn. Peel, trim and slice the carrots and cut the courgettes into approximately 2 cm cubes. Add the vegetables to the pan and cook for another 3–4 minutes. Stir in the cumin powder for a further minute and pour over the water or stock. Bring to the boil and cook on a medium heat for about 30 minutes until all the vegetables are soft. Remove from the heat. Blend the vegetables with a hand blender to smooth. Bring back to the boil then remove from the heat and stir in the basil leaves. Add black pepper to taste before serving.

Handy hint: Use low-salt stock cubes or powder to make stock if you prefer this to plain water. Find them in large supermarkets and health food shops.

Cook's tip: For a richer tasting soup, stir a tablespoon of half-fat crème fraîche or low-fat fromage frais into each bowl of soup immediately before serving.

Grilled aubergine dip

Preparation time:
10 minutes

Cooking time:
15–20 minutes

Fruit/veg per serving:
🍎🍎

This is an easy, tasty and healthy alternative to the shop-bought dips or sandwich fillings. It is great with wraps, pitta bread, low-salt crackers or low-salt tortilla chips or with a baked potato.

Ingredients *(serves 4)*
aubergine • 2 medium
lime • ½, juice only
fresh coriander leaves • 1 handful (approx 20 g), chopped
small onion • ½ small, finely chopped
tomato • 1, seeds removed
cucumber • approx 6 cm chunk (80 g)

Preheat the grill to hot.

Cut the stalk off the aubergines and then slice each in half lengthways. Place cut side down on a lightly oiled baking tray. Grill for about 15–20 minutes or until the skin is blistered and the flesh is very soft. Remove from grill and leave until cool enough to peel the skin off.

Blend the flesh with the lime juice and about half the coriander leaves and half the onion – a hand blender is fine for this, or otherwise just mash well with a fork.

Then chop up the tomato and cucumber – finely or more chunky, as preferred. Stir into the aubergine mixture with the remaining coriander and onion. Serve.

Handy hint: Without the tomato and cucumber the dip will keep for 2–3 days in an airtight container in the fridge. Once the tomato and cucumber have been added, use within 24 hours.

Cook's tip: Try with flat leaf parsley or fresh mint leaves instead of the coriander, and lemon juice instead of the lime, if preferred.

Lemon and coriander houmous

Preparation time:
5 minutes

Cooking time:
5–10 minutes

Fruit/veg per serving:
🍎🍎

So much cheaper, tastier and lower in salt than the shop-bought versions, you can eat this houmous as a starter or snack meal. It will keep for 2–3 days in an airtight container in the fridge.

Ingredients *(serves 4)*

chickpeas in water • 400 g tin (drained)
garlic • 1 small clove, crushed
olive oil • 1 dessertspoon
lemon • 1, juice only
water • 2–4 tablespoons
fresh coriander leaves • 2 tablespoons, finely chopped
freshly ground black pepper
carrots • 4 large, peeled and cut into sticks

Blend the chickpeas, garlic, olive oil and lemon juice with enough water to form a smooth paste, the consistency of thick yoghurt. This can be done with a hand blender, food processor, or even a potato masher. Stir in the coriander leaves and black pepper to taste.

Serve with the carrot sticks or use as a filling for pittas, wraps, sandwiches or baked potatoes.

Handy hint: Feel free to use alternatives to the carrot sticks – try raw cauliflower florets, celery, radish, apple slices and cucumber sticks – the more the better.

Cook's tip: Experiment with different flavours of houmous – try diced red pepper or sundried tomatoes, finely grated carrot mixed in, fresh basil, parsley, dill or a pinch of dried crushed chillies.

Old-fashioned winter soup

Preparation time:
15 minutes

Cooking time:
40 minutes

Fruit/veg per serving:

Filling and warming, this is a meal in itself and a world away from tinned soup. Don't worry about getting the amounts of the vegetables exactly right. Quantities of individual vegetables can be varied, or left out altogether, as long as you include some potatoes and onion. If you don't have swede, try parsnip, turnip or extra carrot instead. Pot barley is a good low GI food to try in soups and stews but if you can't find it, try brown rice instead.

Ingredients *(serves 4)*
onion • 1 large
leek • 1 large
celery • 2 sticks
swede • 100 g piece, peeled
potato • 1 large, peeled
garlic • 1 clove, finely chopped
vegetable oil • 1 tablespoon
pot barley • 50 g
dried red split lentils • 50 g
dried green lentils • 50 g
boiling water • 1.2 litre
bayleaf • 1
black pepper • to taste
low-salt stock cube (optional)
Chinese five-spice powder • ½ teaspoon (optional)

Chop up the onion, leek and celery into small pieces and the swede and potato into 2 cm dice.

Heat the oil in a large, thick-bottomed pan. Add the onion and cook, stirring, over a medium heat for 3–4 minutes, then stir in the leek and celery, swede, potato and garlic. Stir the barley and lentils into the vegetable mixture. Add the boiling water, bayleaf, black pepper (to taste) and a low-salt stock cube, if using.

Bring to the boil, then reduce the heat, cover the pan and simmer for about 40 minutes. Stir occasionally and add hot water if it becomes too thick. Serve piping hot with fresh bread if liked.

Handy hint: Chinese five-spice can be found in most supermarkets. Try using it to boost the flavour of low-salt meat or lentil dishes.

Red onion, thyme and ricotta potato tart

Preparation time:
30 minutes

A delicious vegetarian starter or snack meal. The 'pastry' is easy to make and low in fat and salt.

Cooking time:
35 minutes

Fruit/veg per serving:

Ingredients *(serves 4)*
potatoes • 220 g, peeled
low-fat margarine • 50 g
self-raising flour • 90 g
vegetable oil • ½ tablespoon
red onion • 450 g, finely sliced
garlic • 2 cloves, peeled and crushed
brown sugar • 1 teaspoon
balsamic vinegar • 1 tablespoon
water • 4 tablespoons
fresh thyme leaves • 1 tablespoon
ricotta • 150 g
pine nuts • 20 g

You will need a flan dish, approximately 26 cm diameter, lightly oiled.
Preheat the oven to 200°C/Gas Mark 6.

Boil the potatoes, drain and mash with the margarine. Add the self-raising flour and mix to form a soft dough. Press into the flan dish. Bake for 20 minutes, or until lightly browned.

Meanwhile, heat the oil in a non-stick pan, add the onion and garlic and cook on a low heat for 5 minutes. Add the sugar, balsamic vinegar and water and cook for a further 10 minutes. Remove from the heat, allow to cool slightly and use to fill the pastry case. Dot with teaspoons of ricotta and sprinkle over the pine nuts. Then return to the oven and bake for a further 15 minutes.

Sweet potato, leek and rosemary soup

Preparation time:
5 minutes

Cooking time:
20 minutes

Fruit/veg per serving:
🍎

This tasty version of the standard leek and potato soup makes a filling starter or snack meal. Home-made soups are good low-salt alternatives to the shop bought ones and much cheaper too.

Ingredients *(serves 4)*
vegetable oil • 1 tablespoon
leeks • 2 (approx 300 g)
sweet potato (orange flesh variety) • 1 large
   (approx 400 g)
low-salt stock or water • 500 ml
fresh rosemary, chopped • 1 tablespoon
bayleaf • 1

Peel the sweet potato and cut into approximately 1 cm chunks. Slice the leeks. In a large saucepan heat the oil and add the vegetables. Cook, stirring, for 2–3 minutes. Add the water or stock, the rosemary and the bayleaf. Bring to the boil, then reduce the heat and simmer over a low heat for 20 minutes or until the vegetables are soft. Remove the bayleaf and blend until smooth. If the soup is too thick add a little more boiling water for the preferred consistency.

FISH DISHES

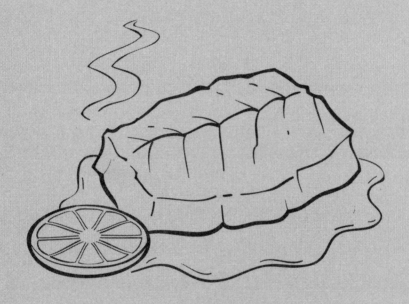

Balsamic fish

Preparation time:
10 minutes

Great for a quick supper, with an easy to make marinade, this will work well with any firm white or oily fish fillets.

Cooking time:
15 minutes

Fruit/veg per serving:
—

Ingredients *(serves 4)*
garlic cloves • 4
white wine • 1 tablespoon
honey • 1 tablespoon
balsamic vinegar • 80 ml
Dijon mustard • 2 heaped teaspoons
oregano • 1 teaspoon
fish fillets • 4 (cod, haddock, salmon or similar)

Preheat the oven to 220°C/Gas Mark 7.

In a small pan, cook the garlic, white wine, honey, vinegar and mustard over a gentle heat for 3 minutes or until thickens slightly. Brush over the fish fillets and bake them in the oven for 15 minutes or until the fish is cooked through. Serve with sweet potato mash or new potatoes and mixed vegetables

Haddock with red pepper sauce

Preparation time:
20 minutes

Cooking time:
20 minutes

Fruit/veg per serving:

🍎🍎🍏

An elegant and easy dish, low in fat and salt, which is perfect for a quick supper or dinner party standby. The couscous and peas are great lower GI accompaniments. Good with most types of fish, including pollock, salmon, cod, plaice and coley. If you don't have fresh coriander, don't worry. Use fresh parsley or chives instead!

Ingredients *(serves 4)*
red peppers • 2 large, seeds and stalk removed
couscous • 200 g
boiling water • 250 ml
frozen green peas • 350 g, defrosted
skinned haddock fillets • 4 (approx 140 g each),
    defrosted if frozen
fresh orange • 4 slices and 2 tablespoons juice
black pepper to taste
olive oil • 2 tablespoons
garlic • 1 clove, crushed
fresh coriander • 1 heaped tablespoon, chopped

Preheat the grill to hot.

Slice each red pepper lengthways into four and grill for 10 minutes or until most of the skin is blackened. Remove the peppers from the grill and put them in a plastic bag or covered plastic container until cool enough to peel the skin away. Then turn the grill down to medium-hot for the fish. Make the sauce by blending together until smooth the peeled red peppers, 1 tablespoon of olive oil, the orange juice, garlic and a couple of grinds of black pepper.

Prepare the couscous by placing in a bowl and pouring over the boiling water. Stir in the peas, cover and leave to stand to absorb all the water. Place the fish fillets in a greased, shallow, heat-proof dish. Top each fillet with a slice of fresh orange and some freshly ground black pepper and drizzle with the remaining tablespoon of olive oil. Grill for approximately 8–10 minutes, depending on the thickness of the fillets, or until the flesh is opaque and flakes easily.

Serve the fish on a bed of couscous and pour any juices in the dish over the couscous. Spoon the warm red pepper sauce over the top. Sprinkle with the fresh coriander.

FISH DISHES

Mackerel with mango salsa

Preparation time:
10 minutes

Cooking time:
8 minutes

Fruit/veg per serving:
🍎

The salsa is an ideal accompaniment to the rich tasting mackerel or other oily fish such as fresh sardines, tuna or salmon. You may prefer to use whole fish, which you can buy cleaned and gutted, but the fillets are easy to use especially if you're not used to handling whole fish. Leave out the chilli if you prefer, or you can use 2–3 drops of Tabasco or similar chilli sauce if this is more convenient.

Ingredients *(serves 4)*
fresh mackerel fillets • 4 medium (or 6–8 small –
    approx 600 g total)

For the salsa
red pepper • ¼
tomato • 1, deseeded
spring onion • 1–2
cucumber • approx 6 cm or 100 g
fresh mango • 1 small
fresh lime or lemon juice • 1 tablespoon
fresh green or red chilli • 1 small, deseeded (optional)

Preheat the grill to hot.

To make the salsa, dice the vegetables and mango and combine together in a bowl with the juice and finely chopped chilli, if using.

Lay the fillets on a lightly greased baking tray, skin side down and grill for about 4 minutes on each side.

Serve the mackerel with a generous spoon of the salsa, boiled rice or new potatoes and a mixed leaf salad or cooked green vegetables.

Pan-fried trout with watercress and walnuts

Preparation time:
15 minutes

A stylish dish, full of heart-healthy ingredients, easy and quick to make as a meal for two or easily halved for one.

Cooking time:
8 minutes

Fruit/veg per serving:
—

Ingredients *(serves 2)*
watercress • 1 bunch (30 g)
red onion • ½ small (30 g), finely sliced
vegetable oil • 1 teaspoon
trout fillets • 300 g, skinned
walnut pieces • 40 g, toasted
crusty bread • 2 thick slices (100 g)

For the dressing
walnut oil or olive oil • 2 tablespoons
sherry or white wine vinegar • 2 tablespoons
maple syrup • 2 tablespoons

First prepare the dressing by whisking all the dressing ingredients together. Alternatively you can put them into a jar with a tight-fitting lid and shake well.

Mix together the red onion and the watercress and divide between two plates. Lightly brush a non-stick pan with oil and cook the fillets over a moderately high heat for about 4 minutes on each side.

On each plate, lay half the trout over the watercress, sprinkle over half the walnuts and then drizzle over the dressing. Serve with the crusty bread or alternatively with boiled new potatoes and a green salad.

Handy hint: Walnuts and other tree nuts are thought to have health benefits but, like most nuts, are relatively high in phosphate and potassium. So you can leave them out if you have been advised to avoid them.

FISH DISHES

Salmon with pea and watercress tagliatelli

Preparation time:
15 minutes

Cooking time:
16 minutes

Fruit/veg per serving:
🍎

A healthy, elegant and delicious dish! Use trout or white fish fillets if you prefer. The tarragon is great with the peas but you can leave it out if you don't have any to hand.

Ingredients *(serves 4)*
fresh salmon • 4 × 150 g pieces
dried tagliatelli • 300 g
frozen peas • 240 g
fresh watercress • 80 g
lemon • 1, juice only
tarragon • 1 teaspoon, dried
   or 1 tablespoon fresh – optional
low-fat cream cheese • 1 generous tablespoon

Preheat the grill to hot.

Place the salmon pieces on a greased, heat-proof dish or tray and grill for 5–8 minutes each side or until just cooked through.

Meanwhile cook the tagliatelli according to the packet instructions and when ready, drain and cover to keep warm.

While the salmon and pasta are cooking make the sauce. Boil the peas for 4-5 minutes. Add the watercress to the pan then drain immediately and then blend until smooth with the lemon juice and tarragon. While the mixture is still warm, stir in the cream cheese and toss the cooked pasta in the sauce.

Serve the salmon on a bed of tagliatelli with a fresh, mixed salad on the side.

Cook's tip: You can use fresh or defrosted frozen spinach instead of the watercress if you prefer and for an alternative serving idea, grill some cherry tomatoes in the tray with the salmon and serve with the finished dish. You could also leave out the pasta and simply serve the sauce with grilled fish, accompanied by boiled new potatoes or couscous and cauliflower, grilled tomatoes or other vegetables.

Spiced salmon

A great spice mix that can be used to add flavour to fish instead of using salt. For a tasty alternative to salmon try using cod, haddock or plaice.

Ingredients *(serves 4)*
garlic clove • 1, crushed
ginger • 1 teaspoon, grated
mild curry powder • ½ teaspoon
cumin • ½ teaspoon
lemons • 2, zest and juice
olive oil • 1 tablespoon
coriander • 1 tablespoon, chopped
salmon steaks • 4

Mix the garlic and ginger together to form a paste. Add curry powder, cumin and lemon juice and zest and mix well. Brush this spice mixture over the salmon and leave to marinate for 10 minutes.

In a non-stick frying pan, fry the salmon in the olive oil on both sides for 3–4 minutes until cooked through. Serve with boiled rice and vegetables or a green salad.

MEAT AND POULTRY

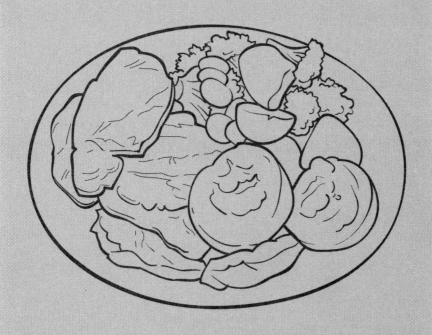

Chicken and sweet potato curry

Preparation time:
15 minutes

Cooking time:
20 minutes

Fruit/veg per serving:

This is a mild curry, which is full of flavour without added salt. It gets its creamy taste from reduced-fat coconut milk, a healthier alternative to standard tinned coconut milk. Don't be put off by the longer list of ingredients – it's fine to use a bought curry powder instead of the individual spices and the curry is so easy and quick to put together that it will be ready in less time than it takes to order in a take-away!

Ingredients *(serves 4)*
rice • 360 g
sweet potato (orange flesh variety) • 2 medium
  (approx 450 g), peeled
sunflower oil • 1 tablespoon
onion • 1 small, chopped
garlic • 2 cloves
cumin powder • 2 teaspoons
coriander powder • 2 teaspoons
turmeric powder • 1 teaspoon
boneless, skinless chicken breasts • 2 large,
  cut into bite-sized pieces
dried red lentils • 4 tablespoons (approx 50 g)
fresh red chilli • 1 medium, seeds removed, finely sliced
low-fat coconut milk • one 400 ml can
water (or low salt stock) • 200 ml
frozen peas • 175 g
pepper • to taste
fresh coriander (optional) • 2 tablespoons, chopped

Cook the rice while the curry is cooking, then drain and keep warm until served.

Cut the sweet potato into approximately 1 cm cubes (larger pieces take too long to cook). In a large saucepan or casserole dish, gently cook the onion in the oil until softened, then add the garlic and spices. Add the chicken breast and sweet potato and stir to coat with the spices. Next add the red lentils, chilli, coconut milk, water or stock and leave to simmer for 15 minutes. Add the peas and simmer for a further 5 minutes.

Serve with the rice, and (if you are using it) sprinkle with the fresh coriander.

Chicken with leek and green bean vinaigrette

Preparation time:
20 minutes

Cooking time:
30 minutes

Fruit/veg per serving:

In this warm salad, plenty of fresh herbs and a tasty vinaigrette dressing provide lots of flavour without the salt. If you can't find fresh tarragon, simply use some extra fresh parsley instead.

Ingredients *(serves 4)*

chicken breasts • 4
olive oil • 100 ml
French green beans • 600 g, trimmed
baby leeks • 16 (or 150 g sliced standard leeks)
Dijon mustard • ½ teaspoon
cider vinegar • 2 tbsp
shallots • 2 chopped
fresh tarragon • 2 teaspoons, chopped
fresh parsley • 4 teaspoons, chopped

Preheat the oven to 180°C/Gas Mark 4. Lightly brush a non-stick frying pan with oil.

Lightly brown the chicken for 2 minutes on each side. Then transfer to an ovenproof dish and bake in the oven for 12–15 minutes until cooked through and the juices run clear.

Meanwhile, trim the leeks and beans and boil for 3 minutes. Then drain and set aside.

To make the salad dressing, mix together the olive oil, mustard and vinegar in a bowl. Cut the leeks and beans diagonally, then add to the dressing with the shallots and herbs.

Place the herby vegetable mixture on a plate, and add the chicken to the top. Drizzle with any remaining salad dressing.

Cook's tip: For a more substantial meal, serve with new potatoes or crusty bread.

Chilli con carne with baked sweet potato

Preparation time:
15 minutes

Cooking time:
30–40 minutes

Fruit/veg per serving:
🍎

Make sure you get the orange fleshed, not the white fleshed, sweet potatoes for this recipe. Obviously you can serve the chilli with rice, standard baked potatoes, bread or another accompaniment but the sweet potatoes and chilli are so good together that even a professional chef didn't spot that there was no salt in his meal!

Ingredients *(serves 4)*
sweet potato (orange flesh) • 4 medium,
    washed but unpeeled
vegetable oil • 1 tablespoon
onion • 1, chopped
garlic • 1 clove, crushed
brown sugar • 1 teaspoon
turkey mince • 450 g
ground cumin • ½ teaspoon
chilli powder • ½ teaspoon
paprika (use smoked paprika if you can
    get it) • 1 teaspoon
tinned tomatoes in rich tomato juice • 400 g tin
tinned kidney beans in water • 400 g tin
fresh coriander leaves (optional) • 1 tablespoon

You will need a medium/large non-stick lidded saucepan.

Preheat the oven to 200°C/Gas Mark 8.

Heat the vegetable oil in the saucepan and cook the onion and garlic with the sugar over a low heat for 5 minutes. Add the turkey mince and cook for a few minutes further, stirring to break up the mince and allow to brown a little. Stir in the spices and then the tomatoes and drained kidney beans. Bring to the boil and then turn the heat down, cover with the lid and allow to simmer for 30–40 minutes. Add a little boiling water if the chilli starts to become too dry.

While the chilli is cooking, place the sweet potatoes on a baking tray or dish. Bake for 30–40 minutes or until cooked through and the flesh is soft.

When the chilli is ready, split the sweet potatoes lengthways and serve with the chilli, a sprinkle of fresh coriander and a mixed leaf salad or boiled/steamed green vegetables.

Colcannon

Preparation time:
20 minutes

Cooking time:
30 minutes

Fruit/veg per serving:

A tried and tested favourite, traditional Colcannon involves lots of ham and lots of butter. This version of the dish keeps the salt and fat levels to a minimum without losing out on taste. Rich in fibre and high in complex carbohydrates this makes for a very satisfying meal.

Ingredients *(serves 4)*

potatoes (desirée or maris piper work best) • 1kg
vegetable oil • 2 tablespoons
semi-skimmed milk • 4 tablespoons
onion • 1 small (sliced)
unsmoked/lower salt bacon • 4 rashers, trimmed of fat
savoy cabbage • 1 medium (500 g), finely sliced
black pepper • to taste
parsley (garnish) • optional

Peel and cut the potatoes into chunks and boil until soft. Drain and mash thoroughly to remove all the lumps. Stir in the olive oil and milk. Season with a few grinds of black pepper.

Meanwhile, fry the onions until soft in the olive oil on a low heat. Grill the bacon. Remove any fat and chop into small pieces. Lastly, boil the cabbage in unsalted water for 3–4 minutes until just cooked. Drain thoroughly before returning it to the pan. Combine onions, bacon and cabbage with the mashed potatoes.

Sprinkle with parsley and serve hot.

Cook's tip: For a vegetarian version of this dish simply omit the bacon. You can add some sliced, unsalted olives if you like.

Handy hints: It's worth taking a closer look at your own favourite recipes. Often some of the fatty or salty ingredients can be reduced, left out or replaced to make a healthier, updated version with all the taste of the original.

Cumin chicken

Preparation time:
10 minutes

Marinating time:
30 minutes

Cooking time:
30 minutes

Fruit/veg per serving:
—

A tasty dish prepared in minutes and low in fat and salt.

Ingredients *(serves 4)*
chicken breasts • 4 (500 g in total)

Marinade
low-fat natural yoghurt • 300 ml
dried coriander or mint • 2 teaspoons
lemon juice • (50 ml)
cumin powder • 1 tablespoon
olive oil • 2 tablespoons
garlic • 2 cloves, crushed

Mix all the marinade ingredients together and rub over the chicken. Leave to marinate in the fridge for at least 30 minutes.

Preheat oven 200°C/Gas Mark 6.

In a hot, non-stick frying pan, seal the chicken on both sides. If your frying pan is not ovenproof, transfer to a lightly-greased ovenproof dish. Bake in oven for 30 minutes until cooked through. Serve with basmati rice and salad.

Honey and ginger lamb

Preparation time:
20–30 minutes

Cooking time:
30–45 minutes

Fruit/veg per serving:
🍎🍎

This great combination of flavours gives the lamb a delicious taste, without the need for salt. Leave out the red chilli if you prefer a milder dish.

Ingredients *(serves 4)*
lamb fillet • 450 g, diced
red pepper • 1
yellow pepper • 1
cherry tomatoes • 100 g
new potatoes • 400 g
mixed salad leaves • 240 g

Marinade
clear honey • 1 generous teaspoon
garlic • 1 small clove
red chilli • 1 small, sliced finely (optional)
ginger • ½ teaspoon, sliced finely
olive oil • 2 tablespoons

Preheat oven to 200°C/400°F/Gas Mark 6.
   Mix the ingredients for the marinade together.
   Stir in the diced lamb, mix well and leave to marinate for 20 minutes. Roast peppers on a baking tray for 20 minutes, then put in plastic bag and allow to cool.
   Meanwhile place lamb in a hot, non-stick frying pan. Cook for 10 minutes until medium rare. While the lamb is cooking, boil the potatoes in water for 15–20 minutes until tender. Remove skin from the peppers and chop them roughly. Toss with tomatoes and potatoes in a large bowl and mix with lamb. Serve with mixed salad leaves.

Jerk pork with pineapple rice

Preparation time:
15 minutes (also needs
a minimum of 1 hour
marinating time)

This recipe uses a delicious combination of herbs and spices to really boost the taste of the meat without adding salt or fat. The meat can be prepared ahead of time and cooked when needed – very convenient when entertaining.

Cooking time:
30 minutes

Fruit/veg per serving:

Ingredients *(serves 4)*
pork loin chops • 4 medium (about 480 g total)

Marinade
onion • 1 small, finely diced
garlic cloves • 2 medium, crushed
ground allspice • 1 teaspoon
dried chilli powder • ½ teaspoon
ground ginger • 1 teaspoon
thyme leaves • 1 teaspoon dried, or 2 teaspoons fresh
vegetable oil • 2 tablespoons
dark rum • 2 tablespoons
lime • 1, juice of

Pineapple rice *(serves 4)*
basmati or long-grain rice • 220 g
spring onion • 4 chopped
red pepper • 1, diced
sweetcorn • 340 g tin in water, drained
    or 200 g frozen, defrosted
tinned pineapple chunks (in juice) • 227 g tin, drained

Blend all the marinade ingredients together to form a smooth paste. Make two or three diagonal slashes in each pork chop. Rub the marinade into the pork. Cover and marinate for at least 1 hour or overnight in the fridge.

Preheat the grill to medium-hot.

Place the chops on a greased, shallow, heat-proof dish. Pour over the remainder of the marinade. Grill the chops for about 10 minutes on each side, or until cooked through. Serve with rice or potatoes and vegetables or the pineapple rice, as follows.

Boil the rice according to the packet instructions. Drain the rice and return to the pan. Stir in the remaining ingredients and heat through.

The rice can also be served with fish, or with grilled or roast meat.

Lemon glazed chicken

Preparation time:
10 minutes

Cooking time:
10 minutes

Fruit/veg per serving:
🍎

This quick, simple and tasty stir-fry takes only a few minutes to make and is free of salt, soy sauce and other salty ingredients.

Ingredients *(serves 2)*
chicken breast • 225 g
vegetable oil • 1 tablespoon
mangetout peas • 140 g
spring onions • 2, finely sliced
water • 2 tablespoons
lemon juice • 2 tablespoons
clear honey • 1 tablespoon
fresh basil leaves • about 1 tablespoon, chopped

Slice the chicken breast into bite-sized pieces. Heat the oil in a large, non-stick pan. Stir fry the chicken for 3–4 minutes until brown. Add the mangetout and spring onions with the water and cook for a further 3–4 minutes. Then add the lemon juice, honey and basil. Leave for a further 1–2 minutes until a glaze has formed and the chicken is cooked through.

Serve with basmati rice as a low-GI accompaniment.

Pasta with a rich bolognese sauce

Preparation time:
20 minutes

This is a rich, delicious sauce. It is packed full of vegetables and flavoured with red wine and herbs instead of salt.

Cooking time:
50 minutes

Fruit/veg per serving:

Ingredients *(serves 4)*
onion • 1 medium
garlic • 2 cloves
celery • 1 stick
carrot • 1 large
vegetable oil • 1 tablespoon
mushrooms • 100 g
dried red split lentils • 40 g
lean minced beef • 300 g
red wine • 200 ml
tinned tomatoes • 1 can (400 g)
tomato purée • 2 tablespoons (approx 40 g)
dried mixed herbs • 2 teaspoons
salt-free stock or water • 100 ml
black pepper • to taste
fresh oregano or flat leaf parsley leaves • 2 tablespoons
dried pasta (white or wholemeal) • 350 g

Finely chop the onion, garlic and celery. Coarsely grate the carrot. Heat the oil in a large saucepan and cook these vegetables over a gentle heat for about 5 minutes, stirring frequently. Slice the mushrooms and add to the mixture with the lentils. Stir in the minced beef, breaking up any lumps and cook for a further 2–3 minutes.

Next add the wine, then the tinned tomatoes, tomato puree, dried herbs, stock and black pepper. Bring to the boil then reduce the heat, cover and cook over a gentle heat for approximately 50 minutes. Check the pan regularly and add more water if the sauce becomes too dry.

Finally, stir in the fresh herbs and serve the sauce with the pasta which has been cooked according to the packet instructions.

Cook's tip: If cooking for 1 or 2 people, make the full amount and freeze any leftovers in portions for convenience. Otherwise, try serving the sauce the next day with baked jacket potatoes, bulgar wheat or bread.

Stuffed cabbage leaves

Preparation time:
30 minutes

Cooking time:
2 hours

Fruit/veg per serving:
🍎🍎🍎🍎

A traditional Eastern European dish which turns some cheap and basic ingredients into a delicious, filling meal. Use beef, turkey or lamb mince if you prefer. You can also use finely chopped or minced leftover cooked meat in place of some or all of the raw meat. Dried mixed herbs can replace the fresh herbs for convenience.

Ingredients *(serves 4)*
chopped tomatoes • 2 medium tins
sugar • 2 teaspoons
lemon • 1, juice only
parsley • 2 tablespoons, chopped
green cabbage • 1 large
onion • 1 small, finely chopped
vegetable oil • 1 tablespoon
minced pork • 150 g
boiled brown rice • 250 g
egg • 1 medium
black pepper • to taste

For the sauce:
Empty the tomatoes into a pan add the sugar and lemon juice and simmer gently for 10–15 minutes. Add the chopped parsley and set to one side.

For the stuffed cabbage leaves:
Meanwhile, remove the outer leaves (you need about 12 in total) from the cabbage. Cut out any thick stalks. Place into boiling water for 1–2 minutes and remove the leaves as they soften. Sauté the onions in the oil to soften and add to the mince, rice and eggs and mix well. Season with black pepper. Place about two tablespoons of the mixture into the centre of a cabbage leaf and roll, tucking in the sides to enclose the filling. Put the meat rolls in a large casserole dish and pour the tomato sauce onto the rolls. Cover with the lid and simmer over a low heat for 2 hours. Check occasionally and add some boiling water if becomes too dry.

Cook's tip: If you prefer, this can also be cooked in a covered casserole dish in a medium oven (180°C/Gas Mark 4) for 1–1½ hours.

VEGETARIAN MAIN DISHES

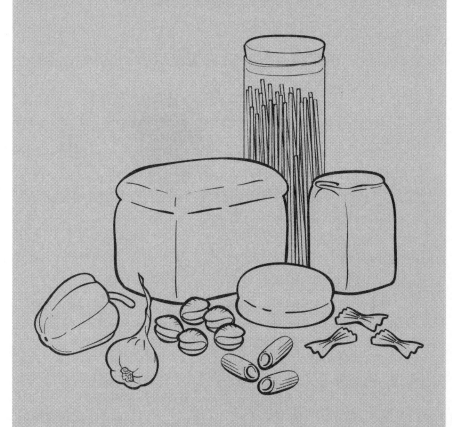

Cannelloni

Preparation time:
35 minutes

Cooking time:
20 minutes

Fruit/veg per serving:
🍎

Give the vegetarian in your life this instead of lasagne and they'll thank you with all their heart! Thanks to the creative wife of a health-conscious (and hungry) GP for passing on this recipe.

Ingredients *(serves 4)*

dried cannelloni tubes or lasagne sheets • 8

For the filling:
ricotta cheese • 250 g tub
frozen chopped (not leaf) spinach • 200 g, defrosted
nutmeg, powdered or freshly grated • ½ level teaspoon
vegetable oil • ½ tablespoon
spring onions • 2–3, finely chopped

For the sauce:
onion • 1
garlic • 1–2 cloves, peeled and crushed
chopped tomatoes • 1 tin (400 g)
tomato purée • 1 tablespoon
bayleaf • 1
dried oregano or mixed herbs • 1 teaspoon
black pepper • to taste
parmesan cheese, grated • 25 g

You will need a medium-sized, ovenproof dish.

For the filling mix the ricotta cheese with the spinach, spring onion, nutmeg, and black pepper to taste. Put aside while you prepare the rest of the dish. This stage can be done up to 24 hours in advance and the mixture kept covered in the fridge until needed.

Next make the sauce. In a medium saucepan, cook the onion in the oil over a gentle heat for 5 minutes or until soft. Add the garlic, tinned tomatoes, tomato purée, herbs, bayleaf and black pepper and cook for about 10 minutes. Remove from heat. Discard the bayleaf before using the sauce.

Fill the cannelloni tubes with the filling mixture. If using lasagne sheets, soften them first in boiling water for about 5 minutes, then use to wrap round the filling to make your own cannelloni tubes.

Continued overleaf

Cannelloni (cont'd)

Take care not to overcook the lasagne as this will make it hard to handle.

Spread half the tomato sauce over the base of the ovenproof dish and place the filled cannelloni tubes on top. Cover with the remainder of the sauce, then sprinkle the parmesan cheese over the dish.

Bake in a pre-heated oven at 180°C/Gas Mark 4 for about 20 minutes or until lightly browned and bubbling.

Serve with a green salad or freshly cooked green vegetables.

Homity pie

Preparation time:
30 minutes

Cooking time:
25 minutes

Fruit/veg per serving:
🍎

This is a variation on the classic vegetarian dish. It is served without the pastry lining and uses mature cheddar to help keep the fat content to an acceptable level without compromising taste.

Ingredients *(serves 4)*

potatoes (desirée or maris piper work best)
  • 2 medium (approx 350 g)
onions • 3 medium (about 450 g), chopped
garlic • 4 cloves, crushed
vegetable oil • 3 tablespoons
mature cheddar cheese • 80 g, grated
semi-skimmed milk • 90 ml
fresh parsley • 1 bunch, chopped
black pepper • to taste

Preheat the oven to 220°C/ Gas Mark 7

Boil or steam the potatoes until tender. Finely chop the onions and garlic and, in a non-stick pan, soften in the oil over a low heat. Combine the potatoes and onions; mix in the remaining oil, parsley, half the cheese, milk and season well with black pepper.

Place in an ovenproof dish. Sprinkle the remaining cheese over the pie, and bake in the oven for about 25 minutes or until golden brown. Serve with some freshly cooked cabbage, carrots, broccoli or preferred vegetable.

Handy hint: Stir in some frozen peas to the mixture before cooking for a colourful and nutritious addition to the dish.

Hot vegetable wraps

Preparation time:
20 minutes

Cooking time:
20 minutes

Fruit/veg per serving:
🍎🍎🍎

Try this for a quick and tasty low-fat lunch or supper dish. The chilli helps boost the flavours of the vegetables without salt, but you can leave it out if you prefer.

Ingredients *(serves 4)*
tortilla wraps • 4
vegetable oil • 1 tablespoon
courgettes • 2 medium
carrots • 2
red pepper • 1
onion • 1 medium
garlic • 1 clove
fresh green or red chilli • 1 small
   (or use ¼–½ teaspoon chilli powder)
tinned chopped tomatoes • 1 small tin
frozen sweetcorn • 80 g (or small tin, drained)
cheddar cheese • 30 g, grated
low-fat fromage frais • 200 ml tub
spring onions • 2, chopped
black pepper • to taste

Preheat the oven to 200°C/Gas Mark 6.

Cut the courgettes, carrots and red pepper into large matchsticks, roughly 3 cm long. Finely slice the onion, garlic and chilli.

In a non-stick pan, heat the oil and stir-fry these vegetables for about 5 minutes – they should still retain some bite.

Warm the tortillas according to the packet instructions. Divide the vegetable mixture between the four tortillas and roll each one up around the portion of vegetables to make the wraps.

Place the wraps in a lightly greased, shallow, ovenproof dish. Mix the chopped tomatoes with the sweetcorn and spread over the wraps. Sprinkle with the grated cheese. Bake in the oven for about 20 minutes or until the cheese is melted and bubbling.

Mix the fromage frais with the chopped spring onion and black pepper to taste. Serve a generous spoonful with the hot wraps, along with plenty of green salad.

Continued opposite

Hot vegetable wraps (cont'd)

Handy hint: The wraps are available in many grocers and supermarkets. They range in salt content so try to choose wraps from the 'healthy eating' ranges, or those with a maximum of 0.3 g sodium per 100 g.

Cook's tip:
You can top the cooked vegetables with some shredded cooked chicken in the wraps if you prefer.

Lentils with spinach

Preparation time:
15 minutes

Cooking time:
35–40 minutes

Fruit/veg per serving:
🍎🍎

This tasty and nutritious store-cupboard standby shows how a few well-chosen flavours liven up some very basic ingredients without the need for salt.

Ingredients *(serves 4)*
onion • 1 medium, finely chopped
garlic • 2 cloves, finely chopped
vegetable oil • 2 tablespoons
carrots • 200 g, diced
celery • 120 g, diced
dried green and/or brown lentils • 200 g
water (or low salt stock) • 600 ml
tinned chopped tomatoes • ½ tin
ground black pepper • ½ teaspoon
fennel seeds • ½ teaspoon
dried thyme • 1 teaspoon
frozen spinach • 200 g
balsamic vinegar • 1 tablespoon
boiled brown rice • 600 g

In a large non-stick saucepan, sauté the onion and garlic in the oil until soft. Stir in the carrots and celery and cook for a further 2 minutes. Add the dry lentils, water and tomatoes, along with the herbs /seasonings.

Bring to the boil. Reduce heat, cover, and simmer for 15–20 minutes. Add frozen spinach. Bring back to the boil and stir to mix thoroughly. Reduce heat, cover, and simmer for another 10–15 minutes until the lentils and carrots are tender.

Stir in the vinegar. Serve with brown rice, chappatis, pitta bread or fresh bread.

Pizza pronto

Preparation time:
20 minutes
plus 30 minutes
proving time

Cooking time:
10 minutes

Fruit/veg per serving:

Think you shouldn't be eating pizza on your healthy diet? Well think again. This one is quick, easy, filling and really tasty but lower in fat or salt than many you might buy in the shops.

If you have a breadmaker, follow the manufacturer's instructions for the base but cut down the salt and add the dried herbs as below. If you only have white flour, cut the water by 20 ml.

If time is really tight, use a bought pizza base, a slice of bread, a halved English muffin or pitta bread. Then add your healthy topping.

Ingredients *(serves 4)*
strong white flour • 200 g
strong wholemeal flour • 200 g
dried fast-acting yeast • 1¼ teaspoons
caster sugar • 1 teaspoon
dried oregano or mixed herbs • 1 teaspoon
salt • ¼ teaspoon
olive oil • 3 tablespoons
warm water • 220 ml

For the topping:
tomato paste • 4 tablespoons
garlic • 4 cloves, finely chopped
dried oregano or mixed herbs • 2 teaspoons
fresh mushrooms • 100 g
onion • 1 medium, finely sliced
low fat mozzarella cheese • 250 g
dried crushed chillies • 1 pinch per pizza (optional)

You will need two large, well-greased baking trays.

Combine the flour, yeast, sugar, herbs and salt in a large bowl. Stir in the oil and the water, making sure that the water feels warm but not hot. Use your hands to combine to a soft dough, adding a little more flour if it is too sticky.

On a well-floured surface, knead the dough for 10 minutes in total.

Continued overleaf·

Pizza pronto (cont'd)

Divide the dough into four pieces and roll out each piece into a circle, approximately 20 cm in diameter. Sprinkle the dough, rolling pin and work surface with flour as required to stop the dough sticking.

Transfer the pizza bases to the baking trays and spread each with a tablespoon of tomato paste. Sprinkle with the garlic and dried herbs. Top with the sliced mushrooms and onion and, lastly, the sliced mozzarella.

Leave in a warm place, out of draughts for 30 minutes to allow the dough to rise. Pre-heat the oven to 220°C, Gas Mark 7.

Bake the pizzas for 10 minutes or until browned and the cheese is bubbling. Serve with a mixed leaf salad. If you like your pizza spicy, sprinkle with some dried crushed chillies to boost the flavour.

Handy hint: If you want to reduce the potassium content of the pizza, use drained, tinned chopped tomatoes in place of the tomato paste. You can also use tinned, sliced mushrooms instead of the fresh mushrooms, or omit altogether.

Other topping ideas:

- Sweetcorn, green and red pepper, sliced fresh green chillies or dried crushed red chillies, cottage cheese and a sprinkling of grated cheddar.

- Spinach, ricotta cheese and pine nuts.

- Frozen mixed roasted vegetables (available from most supermarkets).

- Sliced tomato, fresh basil leaves, low-fat mozzarella.

Quick lentil curry

Preparation time:
15 minutes

Quick, healthy, tasty and easy – what more could you ask for?

Cooking time:
30 minutes

Fruit/veg per serving:
🍎🍎

Ingredients *(serves 4)*
olive oil • 1 tablespoon
ground cumin • 1 teaspoon
ground turmeric • 1 teaspoon
garlic • 1 clove, crushed
pumpkin/butternut squash • 300 g, peeled and cut
  into chunks
new potatoes • 100 g, quartered
chopped tomatoes • 400 g can
brown lentils • 400 g can, drained
fresh coriander leaves • 1 teaspoon, chopped

Heat the oil in large pan. Add the cumin, turmeric and garlic, then cook for 1 minute. Stir in the pumpkin, potatoes and chopped tomatoes. Cover and simmer for 10 minutes.

Add the lentils and cook for further 5 minutes until the potato and pumpkin are cooked. Add coriander and serve with basmati rice, chapattis, pittas or other bread for a speedy meal.

Roasted vegetables with bulgar wheat

Preparation time:
15 minutes

Cooking time:
30–40 minutes

This is inspired by a vegetarian barbecue dish of a friend and colleague who is a great cook (see below). The bulgar wheat is an easy low GI accompaniment which is worth trying, but you can serve the vegetables with pasta shapes, couscous or just bread if you prefer.

Fruit/veg per serving:
🍎🍎

Ingredients *(serves 4)*
pepper, red, yellow or green,
    seeds/stalk removed • 1 large
courgettes • 1 large
aubergine • 1 medium
red onions • 2
fresh herbs
    (rosemary, oregano or thyme) • a large sprig
garlic • 5 cloves, peeled
olive oil • 1 tablespoon
bulgar wheat • 300 g
fresh basil leaves • 2 tablespoons

You will need a large ovenproof shallow dish or roasting tin.

Preheat the oven to 180°C/Gas Mark 6.

Cut the peppers into chunks and thickly slice the courgettes. Cut the aubergine into 1 cm dice. Slice each red onion into about 8 wedges.

Put all the vegetables, the herbs and whole garlic cloves in the ovenproof dish. Drizzle over the olive oil and toss to coat all the vegetables. Roast in the oven for about 30–40 minutes, stirring to turn the vegetables once or twice during the cooking time so that they cook evenly.

Meanwhile prepare the bulgar wheat according to the packet instructions.

Stir the roasted vegetables with all the cooking juices into the cooked bulgar wheat. Stir in the basil immediately before serving.

Cook's tip: This can make a great vegetarian barbeque dish. Keep the peppers and courgettes whole, thickly slice the aubergine lengthways and half the onions. Brush with olive oil and cook the vegetables over the barbecue. Peel the peppers and then cut all the cooked vegetables into bite-sized chunks. Then stir into the bulgar wheat with some crushed garlic and a large handful of basil and/or rocket leaves. Drizzle with some more olive oil and balsamic vinegar.

SIDE DISHES
AND ACCOMPANIMENTS

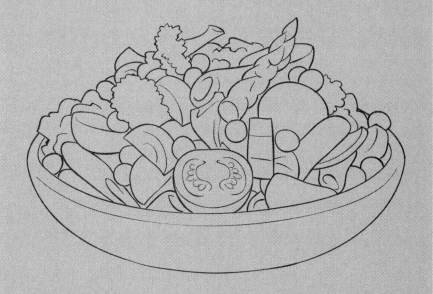

Carrot mashed potatoes

Preparation time:
10 minutes

Cooking time:
20 minutes

Fruit/veg per serving:
🍎

This makes a tasty and colourful mash, and might even persuade reluctant children to eat their vegetables. It works equally well as a side dish, or instead of the standard shepherd's pie topping.

Ingredients *(serves 4)*
potatoes • 300 g
carrots • 350 g
vegetable oil • 1 tablespoon
black pepper • to taste

Peel and trim the potatoes and carrots and cut into chunks. In one large saucepan boil in unsalted water for about 20 minutes or until soft. Drain and mash with the oil and plenty of black pepper.

Cucumber and dill salad

Preparation time:
10 minutes

Fruit/veg per serving:
🍎

Dill is such a delicious herb and goes well with fish. Serve this salad with a piece of grilled fish and new potatoes for a simple, elegant dish for one or more. You won't think twice about leaving out the mayonnaise or other fatty/salty extras.

Ingredients *(serves 4)*
cucumber • 1 large, cubed
fresh dill • 1 heaped tablespoon

For the dressing:
white wine vinegar • 2 tablespoons
sunflower or rapeseed oil • 1 tablespoon
caster sugar • 2 teaspoons
black pepper • to taste

Place the cucumber in a bowl. Mix together the dressing ingredients and pour over the cucumber. Sprinkle with the dill and serve immediately.

Cook's tips:
Buy dill cheaply in bunches from ethnic grocers instead of the supermarket. It also combines well with yoghurt to use as a salad dressing for pasta or potatoes. Otherwise just sprinkle over vegetables such as new potatoes, carrots, mushrooms and green beans.

Finely sliced raw fennel bulb is a good addition to this salad. Find it in good greengrocers and some supermarkets.

No-mayo coleslaw

Preparation time:
10 minutes

A lovely, fresh-tasting salad that is easy and cheap to make all year round.

Fruit/veg per serving:

Ingredients *(serves 4)*
carrot • 1 medium
white cabbage • (approx 200 g)
dessert apple • 1 small, core removed
spring onion • 1–2
low fat plain yoghurt • 3 tablespoons (approx 100 g)
black pepper • to taste
caraway seeds • ½ teaspoon (optional)

Peel, trim and coarsely grate the carrot. Finely shred the cabbage. Cut the apple into small chunks and chop up the spring onion. Combine in a bowl with the yoghurt and black pepper to taste. If you are using the caraway seeds, sprinkle them over the top.

No-salt pesto

Preparation time:
5 minutes

Fruit/veg per serving:
—

Pesto in a jar is a convenient cupboard standby, but it is high in salt. This version is made within a few minutes and is just as tasty.

Ingredients *(enough for 4 portions of pasta)*
pine nuts • 40 g
fresh garlic • 2 cloves
olive oil • 150 ml
fresh basil leaves • 50 g
lemon juice • 20 ml
black pepper • to taste

Place nuts, garlic and olive oil in a blender or food processor and blend for a few seconds to break up the nuts and garlic. Alternatively use a hand blender and allow a little longer. Then add the basil leaves, lemon juice and black pepper and continue to blend until you have a thick, smooth paste. Add more lemon juice and black pepper to taste.

The mixture is ready to use. It keeps well in the fridge with a thin layer of olive oil on top to exclude the air for 3–4 days. You can also freeze it in ice cube trays and have handy portions on standby at any time.

Cook's tips for using the pesto:

- Stir into cooked pasta, roasted vegetables or couscous.

- Drizzle over new potatoes.

- Stir into mashed potato.

- Spread in a toasted sandwich with mozzarella and sliced tomato.

- Toast a wholemeal pitta bread, spread a little pesto inside, then fill with cottage cheese and fresh salad.

- Spread over a fillet of fish, chicken portion or meat chop before grilling or baking it.

- Add a spoonful to pep up some home-made low-salt soup.

Ratatouille

Preparation time:
15 minutes

Cooking time:
50–60 minutes

Fruit/veg per serving:

An easy and invaluable standby that contains all those health-giving vegetables and not much else! Use to top pasta or baked potato, or serve with cold roast meat or grilled fish. It can be eaten hot straight away, or at room temperature. The flavours develop further if it is kept in the fridge (for up to 2–3 days) so you can make it ahead of time. It also freezes well. Don't worry too much about the sizes or weight of the vegetables – a bit of variation is fine.

Ingredients *(serves 4–6)*
olive oil • 2 tablespoons
onion • 1 large, sliced
garlic • 2 cloves, crushed
aubergine • 1 large
courgettes • 4
red pepper • 1 large
tinned tomatoes • 400 g tin
sugar • ½ teaspoon
bayleaf • 1 (optional)
dried oregano or mixed herbs • 1 teaspoon
black pepper • to taste
fresh basil • 1–2 tablespoons (optional)

You will need a large lidded saucepan or casserole, non-stick if possible.

Heat the olive oil in the saucepan or casserole. Add the onion and garlic and cook gently, stirring occasionally, for about 5 minutes until softened. Meanwhile cut the aubergine, courgettes and peppers into chunks (roughly about 2 cm). Add to the pan and stir to coat all the vegetables with the onion mixture. Then add the remaining ingredients, except the basil, to the pan. Cover with the lid and cook on a gentle heat for 45–55 minutes until the vegetables are soft, stirring occasionally. Serve hot or cold, sprinkled with chopped fresh basil leaves if available.

Cook's tip: Serve leftovers cold or hot simply with some couscous, pitta or other bread for a quick snack meal.

Rosemary baked potatoes

Preparation time:
15 minutes

A tasty, low-salt potato dish that is a change from the usual plain roast or boiled alternatives.

Cooking time:
45 minutes

Fruit/veg per serving:

Ingredients *(serves 4)*
olive oil • 2 tablespoons
potatoes • 800 g, thickly sliced
onion • 1 large
garlic • 2 cloves, finely sliced
fresh rosemary • 1 tablespoon, chopped
black pepper • to taste

You will need a casserole or gratin dish.

Using half a tablespoon of the olive oil, grease the casserole dish. In a large pan of boiling water parboil the potato slices for 5 minutes. Meanwhile heat 1 tablespoon of olive oil in a frying pan, add the onions, garlic and rosemary and cook gently over a low heat for approximately 5 minutes or until the onions are softened but not yet starting to brown.

Place a layer of potato slices in the bottom of the dish. Top with a layer of onion mixture and sprinkle with black pepper. Repeat with the rest of the potato and onion mixture, finishing with a neat layer of potatoes.

Drizzle the rest of the olive oil over the top. Bake in a preheated oven at 200°C/Gas Mark 6, for 45 minutes, or until the potatoes are lightly browned and tender.

Serve hot.

Cook's tip: Make ahead of time and then bake in the oven with your roast meat, baked fish or other baked dishes to suit.

Summer butterbean and tomato salad

Preparation time:
10 minutes

Cooking time:
10 minutes

Fruit/veg per serving:
🍎🍎

Ideal for a vegetarian snack meal or as a side dish: the combination of basil with tomatoes is a classic taste of summer. The salad could be made up the night before and taken out in a leak-proof container for a packed lunch or picnic.

Ingredients *(serves 2)*
butterbeans • 1 tin (approx 420 g), drained
tomato • 2 medium, sliced
fresh chives – 1 tablespoon, chopped
olive oil • 1 teaspoon
white wine vinegar • 2 teaspoons
sugar • ½ teaspoon
black pepper • to taste
fresh basil leaves • 2 tablespoons

Mix all the ingredients together except the basil. Tear the basil leaves into small pieces and stir into the salad. Leave to stand for 10 minutes (can be left overnight in the fridge).

Serving suggestion: Serve with bread such as a wholemeal pitta, granary roll or French bread. Could also be mixed with cold pasta or warm boiled new potatoes for a more substantial salad.

Cook's tip: Use kitchen scissors to cut up herbs directly over the dish – it's easier and quicker than using a knife and chopping board.

Traditional red cabbage

Preparation time:
10 minutes

Cooking time:
30 minutes

Fruit/veg per serving:

This practical dish is great with roast poultry, lamb or other meat especially if you are avoiding salty gravy or sauces as it is quite moist. It can also be cooked ahead and then reheated in the oven (or microwave or on the hob) so is perfect to serve with your roast dinner.

Ingredients *(serves 4)*
onion • 1 small
vegetable oil • 2 tablespoons
red cabbage • 250 g approx
eating apple • 1 medium, peeled and cored
wine or cider vinegar • 1 tablespoon
hot water • 2 tablespoons
black pepper • to taste

You will need a lidded saucepan, sauté pan or casserole dish.

Finely slice the onion and cook in the oil over a gentle heat until softened. Finely slice the red cabbage and apple, and add to the onion in the pan. Add the vinegar, water and some black pepper. Cover with the lid and cook over a low heat, stirring occasionally for about 30 minutes or until the cabbage is soft. You may need to add a little more hot water if the cabbage is too dry.

Serve immediately or set aside (or refrigerate if necessary) until needed.

Cook's tip: Try adding a handful of sultanas with the apple (unless you are on a low potassium diet and advised to avoid dried fruit). Fresh, frozen or dried cranberries can be added to serve with your Christmas or Thanksgiving turkey.

DESSERTS

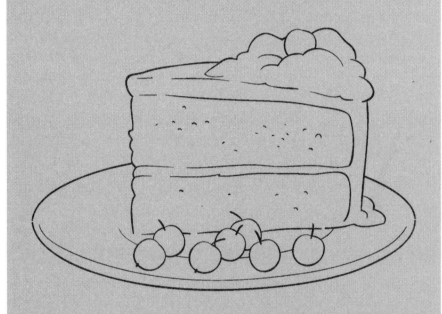

Apple crisps with cinnamon yoghurt dip

Preparation time:
10 minutes

Cooking time:
2+ hours

Fruit/veg per serving:
🍎

For Diabetes:
Reduce sugar content
– see Handy hint

Delicious, crunchy and sweet, these are perfect on their own as a snack or for dipping in plain or flavoured yoghurt, or with ice-cream instead of wafer biscuits. If you are short of time, buy the apple crisps (available in many supermarkets) or use fresh apple slices to serve with the yoghurt dip.

Ingredients *(serves 4)*
sugar • 2 tablespoons
lemon juice • 2 tablespoons
water • 4 tablespoons
crisp eating apples • 2

For the dip:
plain low-fat yoghurt • 400 g
cinnamon • 1 teaspoon

You will need baking trays lined with non-stick paper or heatproof liners.
Preheat the oven to 120°C/Gas Mark ½.

Place the sugar, lemon juice and water in a saucepan and heat gently to dissolve the sugar. Remove from the heat.

Slice the apples very thinly across the width of the apple – a mandolin is useful for this. There is no need to peel or core the apples. Discard the top and bottom slices.

Toss the apple slices in the sugar mixture and then place them in a single layer on the baking trays. Bake for 2 hours until crisp and lightly browned. Then turn off the oven and leave the crisps in the oven until cool. Use immediately or allow to cool completely and store in an airtight container for up to 1 week.

Combine yoghurt and cinnamon to make the dip and serve with the apple crisps.

Handy hint: You can make these without the sugar but they tend to be less crispy and more chewy – in this case, try slicing slightly thicker and baking for 1–2 hours to avoid them getting too dried out.

Cook's tip: Make your own flavoured low-fat yoghurts without artificial colourings or other additives by adding fresh, tinned or frozen fruit. Cinnamon, adds a sweet taste to the yoghurt without needing sugar – or try a drop or two of vanilla essence.

Apple crunch crumble

Preparation time:
15 minutes

Cooking time:
45 minutes

Fruit/veg per serving:
🍎🍎

For Diabetes:
Reduce sugar content
– see Handy hint

More of a crunch than a crumble and the oatey topping is higher in fibre and lower in salt, sugar and fat than the traditional dessert. Best of all – the family will love it!

Ingredients *(serves 6)*
cooking apples • 1 kg
brown sugar • 60 g
mixed spice or cinnamon • 1 teaspoon

For the crunch topping:
porridge oats • 140 g
maple syrup • 70 g
cinnamon • 1 teaspoon
vegetable oil (not olive) • 1½ tablespoons

Peel, core and slice the apples. Put in a saucepan with the sugar and the cinnamon and 2 tablespoons of water. Cook gently for about 15 minutes or until soft. Then transfer to a shallow, ovenproof dish.

Meanwhile, prepare the topping by mixing all the remaining ingredients together. Sprinkle the topping evenly over the apple.

Bake in a preheated oven at 180°C/Gas Mark 4 for 30 minutes or until deep golden brown.

Handy hint: You can use sugar-free sweetener in the apple mixture instead of sugar – refer to the packet instructions.

Blueberry orange muffins

Preparation time:
15 minutes

Cooking time:
15–20 minutes

Fruit/veg per serving:
—

For Diabetes:
Suitable

These are such a good and easy alternative to shop-bought muffins. They are bursting with real fruit rather than artificial flavours, and by selecting a suitable vegetable oil you can make sure that they are free of saturated, trans and other less healthy fats as well as avoiding the salt found in most margarines.

Ingredients *(makes about 12)*
self-raising flour • 270 g
caster sugar • 150 g
skimmed milk • 250 ml
eggs • 2, lightly beaten
sunflower, corn or rapeseed oil • 150 ml
small orange • 1, freshly grated rind only
fresh blueberries • 100 g

You will need a muffin tin, well-greased or lined with paper cases.
Preheat the oven to 220°C/Gas Mark 7.
In a large bowl combine the flour and sugar. Make a well in the centre. In a separate bowl or jug combine the milk, eggs, oil. Add this mixture with the blueberries and orange rind to the dry ingredients. Gently mix together until all the ingredients are only just combined. Be careful not to over-mix – it should look like a lumpy batter.
Divide the mixture between the muffin cases. Bake in the pre-heated oven for about 15–20 minutes or until well risen and lightly browned. Remove the muffins from the tin and leave to cool on a wire rack. They are best eaten the same day but can be kept for a couple of days in an airtight container or freeze well.

Cook's tip: Frozen berries can be used if fresh are not available, or you might like to try using other berries such as raspberries or blackberries. You can also use lemon rind or a teaspoon of vanilla essence to substitute for the orange rind if you prefer.

Cheat's soufflé

Preparation time:
15 minutes

Cooking time:
15–20 minutes

Fruit/veg per serving:
—

For Diabetes:
Caution – reduce
sugar content,
see Handy hint

The exotic fruits combine well in this low-fat dessert. Serve with an extra portion of your preferred fresh or tinned fruit.

Ingredients *(serves 4)*
low-fat custard • 400 ml
icing sugar • 3 teaspoons
limes • zest of 2
passion fruit • 3
egg whites • 3
caster sugar • 1 teaspoon

Preheat oven to 190°C/Gas Mark 5.

Lightly rub the inside of 4 ramekins with oil and sprinkle with the caster sugar. Mix together in a separate bowl the custard, passion fruit, icing sugar and lime zest. In a clean bowl, beat the egg whites until stiff peaks form. Fold lightly into the custard mixture. Spoon into ramekins and bake for 15–20 minutes until puffed up. Do not open the oven door while baking as the soufflés will sink.

Serve immediately with fresh or tinned soft berries, sliced peaches, pear or similar.

Cook's tip: You can prepare ahead by making the custard, fruit and sugar mixture and storing it in the fridge until you are ready to fold in the beaten egg whites.

Handy hint: Shop-bought low-fat custard may not be low in sugar. Make your own with custard powder, semi-skimmed milk and artificial sweetener.

Cinnamon oatmeal muffins

Preparation time:
15 minutes

Cooking time:
20–25 minutes

Fruit/veg per serving:
—

For Diabetes:
Suitable

A handy snack if you are usually too busy to eat breakfast and then get tempted by less healthy foods later in the morning. The oats are a good source of fibre and lower the glycaemic index of the muffin – keeping you fuller for longer. They freeze well so you can keep a stock handy in the freezer.

Ingredients *(makes 12)*
plain flour • 200 g
porridge oats • 60 g
soft brown sugar • 50 g
baking powder • 1 tablespoon
cinnamon • 1 heaped teaspoon
skimmed milk • 250 ml
egg • 1, beaten
oil • 3 tablespoons (30 g)
sultanas • 60 g

Preheat the oven to 220°C or Gas Mark 7.

In a bowl combine the flour, oats, sugar, baking powder and cinnamon. In a measuring jug, measure out the milk and add the oil and beaten egg. Pour this mixture into the bowl with the dry ingredients and stir until just blended. Take care not to over mix. Fold in the sultanas.

Spoon the batter into the prepared muffin tin, dividing evenly. Bake for 20–25 minutes until lightly browned.

Courgette cake

Preparation time:
15 minutes

Cooking time:
1¼–1½ hours

Fruit/veg per serving:
🍎

For Diabetes:
Suitable

Forget carrot cake – this donated recipe is even nicer, really easy and an unusual way to eat your greens! Delicious eaten warm for dessert, or cold at any time.

Ingredients *(for about 10 slices)*
eggs • 2, lightly beaten
caster sugar • 225 g
sunflower, corn or rapeseed oil • 100 ml
courgette • 350 g, grated
self-raising flour • 175 g
chopped nuts • 25 g (optional)
sultanas or raisins • 25 g
vanilla essence • ½ teaspoon
cinnamon or mixed spice • 1½ teaspoons

You will need a 2 lb loaf tin, greased and lined with baking parchment.
    Preheat the oven to 180°C/Gas Mark 4.
    In a large bowl combine all the ingredients and mix well. Pour into the loaf tin. Bake in the pre-heated oven for 1¼ to 1½ hours. Test to see if it is cooked by inserting a clean skewer into the middle of the loaf. If it comes out clean then the cake is done.
    Remove carefully from the tin and leave to cool on a wire rack. Serve warm on its own with stewed fruit, yoghurt or custard as a dessert. Also can be left to cool and eaten as any other cake.

Melon and mint granita

Preparation time:
10 minutes

Cooking time:
4 hours

Fruit/veg per serving:

For Diabetes:
Caution – sugar
content similar
to fruit juice

Like a sorbet, but easier to make, this dessert captures all the flavour of the fruit and is low in fat and calories. It's a good way of using up an overripe melon of any kind – try honeydew, watermelon, or cantaloupe or a mixture.

Ingredients *(6–8 portions)*
ripe melon (any) • 1 kg, rind and seeds discarded
icing sugar • 30 g
lemon juice • 1½ teaspoons
fresh mint leaves • 1 tablespoon, finely chopped

Purée the melon flesh with a hand blender or food processor. Mix in the sugar, the lemon juice and the mint. Pour into a freezer-proof container and freeze for about 1 hour. Stir the mixture to break down the ice crystals and return to the freezer. Repeat hourly for 4 hours in total.

Allow to soften for 20 minutes in the fridge before serving. Serve with fresh strawberries or blueberries when in season.

Orange and mango ice-cream

Preparation time:
15 minutes

A deliciously creamy dessert which is quick and easy to make.

Freezing time:
2 hours

Fruit/veg per serving:
—

For Diabetes:
Suitable

Ingredients *(serves 6–8)*
oranges • 5 large
mango • 2 large, (380 g), stoned and peeled
low-fat natural yoghurt • 50 g
low-fat crème fraîche • 50 g

Grate two tablespoons of rind from one of the oranges. Halve the remaining oranges and scoop out the flesh leaving the skins intact. Put the orange and mango flesh with the orange rind, yoghurt and crème fraîche into a blender. Blend until smooth.

Spoon mixture into a freezer-proof container and freeze for 2 hours, stirring every 15–20 minutes to break up ice crystals. Alternatively, use an ice-cream maker if you have one.

Spoon mixture into empty orange skins, return to freezer for 1 hour, until frozen solid. Allow to soften in the fridge for 30 minutes before serving.

Rum and raisin apple strudel

Preparation time:
20 minutes
(plus 30 mins to soak the raisins)

Cooking time:
40 minutes

Fruit/veg per serving:

For Diabetes:
Suitable, especially
if sugar replaced
by sweetener

Filo pastry desserts are a good choice for home baking as they only contain the fat that you add and there is no rolling or shaping of the pastry. Just handle the sheets gently and make sure you keep the pastry wrapped or covered with a damp cloth to stop it drying out when you are not actually using it.

Ingredients *(makes 2 strudels, or 8 slices)*

raisins • 40 g
rum • 2 tablespoons
cooking apple • 650 g, peeled and cored
soft dark brown sugar • 100 g
cinnamon • ½ teaspoon
mixed spice • 1 teaspoon
mixed citrus peel • 25 g
filo pastry • 8 small sheets
vegetable oil • 2 tablespoons

You will need a large baking tray lined with baking parchment.

Mix the raisins with the rum and leave to soak for at least 30 minutes. Preheat the oven to190°C/Gas Mark 5.

Cut the apple into small, thin slices. Add the raisins and rum, the sugar, spices and mixed peel and mix well.

Lay one filo pastry square on the work surface and using a pastry brush, dab all over with a little of the oil. Place a second pastry square on top of the first and again dab with the oil. Repeat this twice more.

Spread half the apple mixture all over the filo pastry, leaving a 2 cm border all round. Fold in the border of the two long sides over the apple mixture. Then, starting from one of the short sides, roll up the pastry to enclose the apple mixture (just like a Swiss roll). Place the rolled-up strudel on the baking tray, making sure that the end of the pastry sheet is hidden underneath the roll. Repeat with the remaining pastry sheets and apple mixture to make a second strudel. Brush all over with any remaining oil. Bake for 40 minutes or until lightly browned.

Serving suggestion: Serve hot for dessert with low-fat plain fromage frais or custard made with semi-skimmed milk (and artificial sweetener if you prefer). Otherwise, leave to go cold and keep in the fridge if you prefer. A slice goes well with a cup of tea or coffee.

Summer fruit terrine

Preparation time:
10 minutes

Chill time:
4 hours

Fruit/veg per serving:
🍎

For Diabetes:
Suitable

This is a great dessert for dinner parties and can be made in advance. You can use either fresh or frozen berries. It is also a good way to get fruit into children!

Ingredients *(serves 4–6)*
sugar-free jelly • sufficient to make up 580 ml
frozen summer fruits (or seasonal fresh berries)
• 350 g, defrosted
low-fat fromage frais • 1 heaped tablespoon

Line a small loaf tin with clingfilm. Make up the jelly as directed. Put the defrosted berries in the bottom of the tin and pour over the liquid jelly.

Leave to set in fridge for 4 hours, then turn out onto a plate and serve in slices with a spoonful of fromage frais.

Summer pudding

Preparation time:
30 minutes

Cooking time:
4 hours

Fruit/veg per serving:
🍎

For Diabetes:
Suitable

A tasty, fruity, low-sugar, low-calorie pudding that can be prepared ahead of time. Use frozen berries as the juice is used to soak the bread.

Ingredients *(serves 4)*
white bread • 8 slices (approx 200 g), with crusts
  removed
frozen mixed summer berries • 350 g, defrosted
artificial, granulated sweetener • 1 tablespoon

You will need 4 individual ramekin dishes, teacups or similar (they do not need to be heat-proof).

Defrost the fruit thoroughly, strain off juice into a bowl and reserve. Add the sweetener to the fruit. Take half the bread and cut each slice into half and then into strips to fit your mould. Take the other half of the bread and, using a ramekin dish as a guide, cut out two circles to fit top and bottom for each of the four ramekin dishes. Dip the strips and circles of bread in the juice and line each of the ramekin dishes. Use the bread trimmings to fill in any gaps. Put a quarter of the fruit into each ramekin and top with the second circle of bread. Cover with clear film wrap and weigh down with plate.

Leave to chill in fridge for 4 hours or overnight. Turn out and serve with low-fat fromage frais or yoghurt.

Upside-down lemon cheesecake

Preparation time:
10 minutes

Chilling time:
2–3 hours or overnight

Fruit/veg per serving:
—

For Diabetes:
Caution: high
sugar content

A new take on the traditional cheesecake: delicious with a portion of your favourite fruit.

Ingredients
(serves 4)

quark (or very low-fat cream cheese) • 250 g
lemon curd • 80 g
ginger biscuits • 40 g

You will need four individual ramekin dishes or similar.

Mix together lemon curd with quark. Split between 4 ramekins. Break biscuits into fine breadcrumbs and sprinkle over the top of each ramekin. Place in the refrigerator to chill for at least 2–3 hours, and overnight if possible.

Serve with fresh summer berries or other preferred fresh, frozen or tinned fruit.

APPENDICES

Appendix 1
Useful addresses and websites

National Kidney Federation
The Point
Coach House
Shireoaks
Worksop
Notts S81 8BW
Tel: 01909 544999
Fax: 01909 401723
Helpline: 0845 601 02 09
Website: www.kidney.org.uk

Kidney Research UK
King's Chambers
Priestgate
Peterborough
PE1 1FG
Tel: 0845 070 7601
Helpline: 0845 300 14 99
Email: info@kidneyresearchuk.org
Website: www.kidneyresearchuk.org

Nephronline
Website: www.nephronline.org
Gives information on various aspects of kidney disease and CKD, including specialist advice on dietary issues.

The Food Standards Agency
Website: www.eatwell.gov.uk
Government Department's dietary information page aimed at the person who wants to choose a healthy diet.

The Marine Stewardship Council
Website: www.fishonline.org/advice/eat
Provides information on where to buy fish from sustainable sources.

Diabetes UK
10 Parkway
London
NW1 7AA
Tel: 020 7424 1000
Fax: 020 7424 1001
Helpline: 0845 120 29 60
Website: www.diabetes.org.uk

The British Dietetic Association
5th Floor
Charles House
148–9 Great Charles Street
Queensway
Birmingham
B3 3HT
Tel 0121 200 8080
Fax 0121 200 8081
Website: www.bda.uk.com

British Heart Foundation
14 Fitzhardinge Street
London
W1H 6DH
Tel: 020 7935 0185
Fax: 020 7486 5820
Website: www.bhf.org.uk

Appendix 2 – Nutritional analysis of recipes per portion

Recipe	Per portion						Per 100 g
	Calories kCal	Protein g	Fat g	Saturated fat g	Potassium mg	Phosphorous mg	Sodium mg
Apple crisps with cinnamon yoghurt dip	131	5	1	1	339	151	29
Apple crunch crumble	245	4	6	0	379	103	9
Baked tomatoes	140	5	5	1	669	127	70
Balsamic fish	126	19	2	0	395	204	123
Blueberry orange muffins	261	4	14	2	86	141	121
Cannelloni	314	17	12	6	762	292	49
Carrot mashed potatoes	100	2	3	0	315	38	30
Cheat's soufflé	123	6	2	1	241	125	92
Chicken and sweet potato curry	402	28	5	1	1158	368	33
Chicken with leek and green bean vinaigrette	410	35	28	4	870	370	27
Chilli con carne with baked sweet potato	467	37	5	1	1874	502	86
Cinnamon oatmeal muffins	146	4	4	1	143	155	229
Colcannon	360	15	13	3	1249	211	84
Courgette and carrot soup	111	3	6	1	506	66	7
Courgette cake	281	4	13	2	216	130	87
Cucumber and dill salad	46	1	3	0	135	42	4
Cumin chicken	230	34	8	2	719	402	57
Grilled aubergine dip	28	2	1	0	384	39	3
Haddock with red pepper sauce	435	38	8	1	958	442	23
Homity pie	280	10	16	6	580	199	63
Honey and ginger lamb	400	25	22	8	946	285	22
Hot vegetable wraps	336	15	6	1	792	248	75
Jerk pork with pineapple rice	532	34	11	2	801	384	69

Lemon and coriander houmous	138	5	5	1	311	72	84
Lemon glazed chicken	231	30	7	1	620	299	31
Lentils with spinach	465	19	9	2	1176	420	12
Mackerel with mango salsa	357	29	24	5	584	324	41
Melon and mint granita	51	1	0	0	269	21	31
No-mayo coleslaw	43	2	1	0	239	57	22
No-salt pesto	1657*	8*	178*	23*	575*	302*	2*
Old-fashioned winter soup	224	10	4	0	746	179	7
Orange and mango ice-cream	82	2	2	1	258	45	9
Pan-fried trout with watercress and walnuts	624	38	35	4	879	496	116
Pasta with a rich bolognese sauce	550	32	9	2	1229	421	30
Pizza pronto	557	24	18	7	739	402	131
Quick lentil curry	132	8	4	1	662	128	17
Ratatouille	138	5	7	1	997	112	11
Red onion, thyme and ricotta potato tart	313	10	15	4	489	266	77
Roasted vegetables with bulgar wheat	360	11	5	1	795	326	3
Rosemary baked potatoes	219	5	6	1	673	83	6
Rum and raisin apple strudel	179	2	4	0	168	26	48
Salmon with pea and watercress tagliatelli	496	35	14	3	743	474	30
Spiced salmon	208	21	14	2	409	258	40
Stuffed cabbage leaves	279	15	10	3	1076	277	24
Summer butterbean and tomato salad	124	8	2	0	564	103	237
Summer fruit terrine	35	4	0	0	221	46	7
Summer pudding	148	6	1	0	235	76	200
Sweet potato, leek and rosemary soup	132	3	4	1	587	86	14
Traditional red cabbage	81	1	6	1	216	31	5
Upside-down lemon cheesecake	146	10	2	1	112	137	80

* Total recipe value as portions vary.

All nutrient analyses in the table on pages 142–3 have been calculated using Dietplan6 with additional data from the USDA website (United States Department of Agriculture – www.usda.gov). They are based on food weight and food selection according to available data, recipe specification or standard food portion sizes as defined in *Food Portion Sizes*, 2nd edition, by the Ministry of Agriculture, Fisheries and Food, 1993). It should be borne in mind that food portions served at home are likely to vary slightly in size, but every effort has been made to be as accurate within this limitation.

Index

Feedback Form

We hope that you found this *Class Health* book helpful. We always appreciate readers' opinions and would be grateful if you could take a few minutes to complete this form for us.

❶ How did you acquire your copy of this book?

From my local library ☐

Read an article in a newspaper/magazine ☐

Found it by chance ☐

Recommended by a friend ☐

Recommended by a patient organisation/charity ☐

Recommended by a doctor/nurse/advisor ☐

Saw an advertisement ☐

❷ How much of the book have you read?

All of it ☐

More than half of it ☐

Less than half of it ☐

❸ Which chapters have been most helpful?

....

....

❹ Overall, how useful to you was this *Class Health* book?

Extremely useful ☐

Very useful ☐

Useful ☐

❺ What did you find most helpful?

....

....

❻ What did you find least helpful?

....

....

❼ Have you read any other health books?

Yes ☐   No ☐

If yes, which subjects did they cover?

....

....

....

How did this *Class Health* book compare?

Much better	☐
Better	☐
About the same	☐
Not as good	☐

❽ Would you recommend this book to a friend?

Yes ☐   No ☐

Thank you for your help. Please send your completed form to:

Class Publishing, FREEPOST, London W6 7BR

Surname   First name
_____

Title Prof/Dr/Mr/Mrs/Ms
_____

Address
_____

_____

Town   Postcode   Country
_____

☐ Please add my name and address to receive details of related books
[*Please note, we will not pass on your details to any other company*]

Have you found **Eating Well for Kidney Health** *useful and practical?*
If so, you may be interested in other books from Class Publishing.

Kidney Failure Explained
Dr Andy Stein and Janet Wild   £17.99

This fully updated new edition of the complete reference manual that gives you, your family and friends, the information you really want to know about managing your kidney condition. Written by two experienced medical authors, this practical handbook covers every aspect of living with kidney disease – from diagnosis, drugs and treatment, to diet, relationships and sex.

> '. . . *remains the most sought after reference for kidney patients.*'
> **Timothy F Statham OBE**
> Chief Executive
> the National Kidney Federation

Eating Well with Kidney Failure
Helena Jackson, Annie Cassidy
and Gavin James   £14.99

If you have kidney failure, you need to adapt and change what you eat. But, as this practical and exciting new book shows, you don't need to go on a crash diet, or deny yourself the foods you love – you just need to adapt your favourite recipes with kidney-friendly foods.

The authors have provided more than fifty delicious recipes to show you how this works in practice. The recipes have been analysed for their nutritional content and are coded to help you choose the most appropriate dishes for your individual requirements.

Dump Your Toxic Waist!
Lose inches, beat diabetes and stop that heart attack
Dr Derrick Cutting   £14.99

The easy, drug-free and medically accurate way to cut dramatically your risk of having a heart attack. Even if you already have heart disease, you can halt and even reverse its progress by following Dr Cutting's simple steps. Don't be a victim – take action now!

> '*Highly recommended.*'
> **Michael Livingston**
> Director
> HEART UK

Type 1 Diabetes:
Answers at your fingertips

Type 2 Diabetes:
Answers at your fingertips
Dr Charles Fox and Dr Anne Kilvert
£14.99 each

The latest edition of our bestselling reference guide on diabetes has now been split into two books covering the two distinct forms of the disease. These books maintain the popular question and answer format to provide practical advice on every aspect of living with the condition.

> '*I have no hesitation in commending this book.*'
> **Sir Steve Redgrave**
> Vice President
> Diabetes UK

High Blood Pressure: Answers at your fingertips

Dr Tom Fahey,
Professor Deirdre Murphy
with Dr Julian Tudor Hart   £14.99

The authors use all their years of experience as blood pressure experts to answer your questions on high blood pressure, in order to give you the information you need to bring your blood pressure down – and keep it down.

> '*Readable and comprehensive information.*'
> **Dr Sylvia McLaughlan**
> Director General
> The Stroke Association

Stroke: Answers at your fingertips

Dr Anthony Rudd, Penny Irwin
and Bridget Penhale   £17.99

This essential guidebook tells you all about strokes – most importantly how to recover from them. As well as providing clear explanations of the medical processes, tests, and treatments, the book is full of practical advice, including recuperation plans. You will find it inspiring.

> '*If you only buy one book about stroke, it should be* Stroke: Answers at your fingertips.'
> **Jon Barrick**
> Chief Executive
> The Stroke Association

Beating Depression

Dr Stefan Cembrowicz
and Dr Dorcas Kingham   £17.99

Depression is one of the most common illnesses in the world, affecting up to one in four people at some time in their lives. This book shows sufferers and their families that they are not alone, and offers tried and tested techniques for overcoming depression.

> '*All you need to know about depression presented in a clear, concise and readable way.*'
> **Ann Dawson**
> The World Health Organization

Kidney Transplants Explained

Dr Andy Stein, Dr Rob Higgins
and Janet Wild   £17.99

A successful kidney transplant can transform the life of a person with kidney failure and people with a well-functioning transplant often feel much fitter than they did on dialysis. Not everyone is suitable for transplant however, and those who are may not be suitable all of the time.

If you need a kidney transplant, it is essential to be thoroughly prepared. This book will help you by answering your questions about transplants and what they involve. Indispensable to people considering a transplant or already living with one, this guide will also be valuable for anyone considering kidney donation.

> '*I wish I'd had access to a similarly intelligent book when I first encountered kidney failure 20 years ago.*'
> **Deborah Duval**
> Editor, *Kidney Life*

PRIORITY ORDER FORM

Cut out or photocopy this form and send it (post free in the UK) to:

Class Publishing Priority Service
FREEPOST 16705
Macmillan Distribution
Basingstoke RG21 6ZZ

Tel: 01256 302 699
Fax: 01256 812 558

Please send me urgently
(tick boxes below)

Post included
price per copy (UK only)

☐ **Eating Well for Kidney Health** (ISBN 9781859592045)	£17.99
☐ **Eating Well with Kidney Failure** (ISBN 9781859591161)	£17.99
☐ **Kidney Failure Explained** (ISBN 9781859591451)	£20.99
☐ **Dump Your Toxic Waist!** (ISBN 9781859591981)	£17.99
☐ **Type 1 Diabetes: Answers at your fingertips** (ISBN 9781859591758)	£17.99
☐ **Type 2 Diabetes: Answers at your fingertips** (ISBN 9781859591765)	£17.99
☐ **High Blood Pressure: Answers at your fingertips** (ISBN 9781859590904)	£17.99
☐ **Stroke: Answers at your fingertips** (ISBN 9781859591130)	£20.99
☐ **Beating Depression** (ISBN 9781859591505)	£20.99
☐ **Kidney Transplants Explained** (ISBN 9781859591932)	£20.99

TOTAL _____

Easy ways to pay

Cheque: I enclose a cheque payable to Class Publishing for £ _____

Credit card: Please debit my   ☐ Mastercard   ☐ Visa   ☐ Amex

Number _____ Expiry date _____

Name _____

My address for delivery is _____

_____

Town _____ County _____ Postcode _____

Telephone number (*in case of query*) _____

Credit card billing address if different from above _____

_____

Town _____ County _____ Postcode _____

Class Publishing's guarantee: remember that if, for any reason, you are not satisfied with these books, we will refund all your money, without any questions asked. Prices and VAT rates may be altered for reasons beyond our control.

$$3.14$$
$$4$$
$$2 \overline{)12.46}$$
$$6.23$$